Memorize

For PG Entrance Examination

A must-buy for NEET, PGI, AIIMS, FMGE, and JIPMER entrance exams

• Anatomy • Embryology • Histology • Physiology • Biochemistry • Microbiology • Pathology • Pharmacology • Forensic Medicine • Social and Preventive Medicine • Biostatistics • ENT • Ophthalmology • General Medicine • Surgery • Obstetrics and Gynecology • Pediatrics • Psychiatry • Dermatology • Orthopedics • Radiology • Anesthesiology

Memorize
For PG Entrance Examination

Author

Dhileepan Selvarajan MD
(Gold Medalist)
Resident Physician
Department of Internal Medicine
Cleveland Clinic Akron General Hospital
Akron, Ohio, USA
Formerly Assistant Professor of Medicine
Vinayaka Mission's Medical College
Karaikal, Puducherry, India

Co-Authors

Vidyasagar Ramalingam MD
All India Institute of Medical Sciences (AIIMS)
Delhi, India

Vishwanath Iyer MD
National Institute of Mental Health & Neurosciences (NIMHANS)
Bengaluru, Karnataka, India

JAYPEE *The Health Sciences Publisher*
New Delhi | London | Philadelphia | Panama

JAYPEE Jaypee Brothers Medical Publishers (P) Ltd

Headquarters
Jaypee Brothers Medical Publishers (P) Ltd.
4838/24, Ansari Road, Daryaganj
New Delhi 110 002, India
Phone: +91-11-43574357
Fax: +91-11-43574314
E-mail: jaypee@jaypeebrothers.com

Overseas Offices
J.P. Medical Ltd.
83, Victoria Street, London
SW1H 0HW (UK)
Phone: +44-20 3170 8910
Fax: +44(0)20 3008 6180
E-mail: info@jpmedpub.com

Jaypee-Highlights Medical Publishers Inc.
City of Knowledge, Bld. 235, 2nd Floor, Clayton
Panama City, Panama
Phone: +1 507-301-0496
Fax: +1 507-301-0499
E-mail: cservice@jphmedical.com

Jaypee Medical Inc.
325 Chestnut Street
Suite 412
Philadelphia, PA 19106, USA
Phone: +1 267-519-9789
E-mail: support@jpmedus.com

Jaypee Brothers Medical Publishers (P) Ltd.
17/1-B, Babar Road, Block-B, Shaymali
Mohammadpur, Dhaka-1207
Bangladesh
Mobile: +08801912003485
E-mail: jaypeedhaka@gmail.com

Jaypee Brothers Medical Publishers (P) Ltd.
Bhotahity, Kathmandu, Nepal
Phone: +977-9741283608
E-mail: kathmandu@jaypeebrothers.com

Website: www.jaypeebrothers.com
Website: www.jaypeedigital.com

Inquiries for bulk sales may be solicited at: jaypee@jaypeebrothers.com

Memorize: For PG Entrance Examination

First Edition: **2017**

ISBN: 978-93-86150-78-3

Printed at Sanat Printers

Dedication

I dedicate this book to my parents and family
My father—N Selvarajan
My mother—V Kalaichelvi
My sister—S Jegan Kuttimani
My brother—S Prabakaran

Dhileepan Selvarajan

Preface

Memorize is the product of three years of sheer hard work of three doctors who are high rank holders in all entrance examinations and have been shining in their fields. Memorize is mainly for the last minute revision. It is not advisable to read this book while start preparing as this is so concised and highly concentrated subject. We prepared this book in the view of candidates not missing objective answers and those need use of memory. This also equips us with analyzing some tougher questions.We have prepared this book from a student point of view so that it is easy for their preparation.

This book will be helpful to face not only NEET examination but also AIIMS, JIPMER, PGI and all state entrance examinations. Each word in this book is so important as they are collected from various sources. It contains more precise things and will give definitely an edge if it is read. If this book is read, definitely will give 20% marks extra.

Dhileepan Selvarajan MD

Acknowledgments

First of all I convey my heartful thanks to the co-authors Dr Vishwanth Iyer and Dr Vidhyasagar Ramalingam who helped me in typing and contributing to this book. I would like to convey my sincere thanks to Mr Jayananthan of Jaypee Brothers Medical Publishers (Chennai) who has motivated me to write this book and got the approval. At this juncture I wish to thank my mentor Dr Chenniappan who is the "Teacher of Teachers" who inspired me in the field of medicine. I also thank Dr Noorul Ameen, Dr Vasanthi and Dr Muralitharan for their support. I specially thank to Dr Suhasini for helping me in writing radiology and Dr Barath for SPM. I also convey my gratitude to my friends Dr Ramesh, Dr Jeyabalaji, Dr Praveen, Dr Janakiraman and Dr Vanitha for their moral support.

Exam Tips

"Now, here, you see, it takes all the running you can do, to keep in the same place."

– Red Queen in Lewis Carroll's Through the Looking-Glass

Also called the ***"Red Queen Hypothesis"*** in evolutionary biology, this statement holds good for our postgraduate medical entrance examinations. Some even go to the extent of considering these exams as "a rat race" for doctors. Problems appear daunting to us only when we know the issues but with none of the steps to solve them. A systematic approach will help us understand the steps necessary to solve any kind of task.

STEP BY STEP

Prior to Exam

One can start, say years before, months before or even weeks before an exam. The time needed for the preparation varies from person to person, exam to exam, and also the target expected to achieve. However, it is always safe to target the best possible results and start as early as possible.

Now that said, an undergraduate student can start right away and try to finish the standard textbooks in the coursework and use entrance exam-oriented books as an assistance. An intern can try and devise an intensive exam-oriented plan whenever time permits. In post MBBS, one can try an intensive exam-oriented preparation with retrograde textbook assistance. And always remember: "It is never too late." So, the first keyword is: **"START!"**

Here the focus will be on intensive exam-oriented preparation. Choose the set of books you are planning to finish, depending on the time available for preparation, and choose wisely! It is always better to start with subjectwise entrance books. Classify the subjects into large, medium-sized, and small, and allot time accordingly (e.g. Medicine, Surgery, PSM as large; Ophthalmology, ENT, Pediatrics as medium; Skin, Anesthesia, Radiology as small). Some may choose to join classes or residential programs while some may choose to study at home or in a library. Also some may prefer individual study while some may prefer group study. Whatever method you choose to follow, remember to **"COVER ALL SUBJECTS"**, and do not compromise on this point.

Each subject carries different weightage in different exams and it also varies from year to year (e.g. AIIMS gives more weightage to clinical subjects, PSM and—for some strange reason—Ophthalmology, while NEET pattern generally gives equal weightage preclinical and clinical subjects; whereas, for PGI, molecular biology is important). Nevertheless, one thing I noticed, while I attended my exams and from the experience of friends and seniors, that preclinical and, to some extent, paraclinical subjects played a major role in making the difference between the toppers and others. This may be due to the fact that students tend to forget a major chunk of basic science subjects learnt long back. Hence, **NEVER MISS THE BASIC SCIENCES**.

The initial study would consume the major part of the time, almost two-third of the study duration. However, the most important part is the remaining one-third, which is **REVISION**. During the initial study, it is recommended that one should make notes of the subjects in a separate notebook or at least highlight the important points and points that one tends to forget. This should be in such a way that the entire study material is reduced to at least one-tenth the original size (the smaller the better) and one should use this for revision. Also take the aid of concise revision books which cover all the subjects. Revise as many times as possible, at least twice. The questions which we tend to mark wrongly are the ones which play the major role in making a difference in the score. So, strive to get this right by revision. Note these questions by marking them or by maintaining a log of these questions. Never should you forgive yourself for missing these questions when repeated in exams. So, get all the repeat questions and topics correct to **EVEN STAY IN THE SAME PLACE**. So, this is the hard work part, and the rest of the difference is created by **PROPER STRATEGY**.

While studying, **MAKE ALL THE CONCEPTS CLEAR**. Concepts once made clear are rarely forgotten. However, not all topics or questions involve concepts, and several topics may require rote learning. Memory can fail anyone. So, use memory aids, such as mnemonics (mnemonics which are as funny as possible and which you can easily remember), make mind maps, diagrams (would also help solve picture questions asked nowadays, flashcards or simply teach someone)! Get pics (mobile camera comes handy here) of flowcharts or tables from standard books and keep reviewing them in your spare time. Get adequate rest; take scheduled breaks so that what you study stays in mind. Some amount of stress is good, but there is a very thin line between stress that is positive and stress that pulls you down. Hence, use stress-busters which work for you—music, walk, talk, TV, whatever. At the end of the day, make learning an enjoyable experience!

EXAM DAY

Exam day is the most important day, as your performance given on the day is the culmination of all efforts. Do not spoil the day by capricious instances, such as forgetting something that is needed for the exam or arriving late for the exam. Do all it takes to maintain your composure for a clear thought process.

The usuals

Read the question statements and options fully, do not miss parts like most common, all except, not... least likely, etc., do not spend too much time on a single question; the questions that take up a lot of your time are usually the ones which you are going to get wrong; for difficult stuff, let your subconscious do the work while you go about answering the remaining ones; stick to the time while answering questions (prior practice helps here); allot time for revising or revisiting difficult questions; rest your eyes once in a while if you are sitting for an online exam; for OMR-based exams, see whether you are marking answers for the appropriate questions and that you are not skipping rows; for online exams, ensure that you save your answers, if that is required.

Now to some unconventional stuff

An important problem faced by students is the number of questions to attend when there are negative markings. Simple—**PLAY BY RULES–PLAY WITH PROBABILITY**. Consider an example: there are 200 questions with +1 for the right answer and –1/3 for the wrong answer. If you answer everything by chance, you have 1/4 chance of getting a right answer and chance of getting a wrong answer. Mathematically, you would end up getting $+1 \times 1/4 - 1/3 \times 3/4 = 0$. Even if you can rule out one option for a question, the probability works in your favor. This is the usual scenario that in a paper of 200 questions, for around 100 questions, you would know one right answer, for another 60 or more questions, you would be able to rule out 2 options and for another 30 or more questions, you may be able to rule out at least 1 option. So, in this manner, you would be able to attend most of the questions, except for a few factual or numerical or totally unheard-of questions, i.e. around 190+ questions.

More tricks

Allot time for initial solving of questions and for revisiting (once or twice) questions. You would gain a lot of detail in the initial run; for instance, some themes get repeated in more than one question and identifying them may help solve some questions, which would have otherwise been unsolvable. You may get a rough idea about the subjectwise distribution of questions and subconsciously recognise what subject a question and, hence, the answer belong to. Also you would know how many As, Bs, Cs or Ds you have marked (an exam wouldn't have only Bs!) or the number of options you have marked—in case of PGI. Get into the examiner's shoes and think as an examiner would think. Many a times, this yields an answer to vague questions. Whenever there are two contradictory options, usually one of them is the answer. The lengthier an option is framed, the more the chances that the examiner has tried to make it an answer. However, the more the number of statements or assertions made in a single option, the more are the chances that one of them is wrong and, hence, the option could be the answer for an "all except" question. Remember that each option has been given for a reason; very rarely are the totally unrelated or irrelevant statements given as options. Think twice before marking option A as an answer. Few examiners would tend to provide the answer in the first option. However, when the exam involves computerized randomization of options (very likely), this method would not work. Neither are these fool-proof methods, nor are they part of routine answering—they may simply be of help **WHEN YOU DON'T KNOW THE ANSWER!**

Contents

CHAPTER 1

Anatomy

EPITHELIUM

Simple squamous	***Endothelium*** ***Mesothelium*** ***Ascending thin loop of henle, Endocardium***
Simple cuboidal	***Collecting duct, DCT, PCT*** ***Respiratory bronchioles*** ***Rete testis and tubuli recti*** ***Ovary*** ***Ependyma***
Simple columnar **Ciliated** **Non-ciliated**	 ***Fallopian tube, endometrium, central canal*** ***Stomach, small and large Intestine, GB, bulbourethral glands and ejaculatory duct***
Stratified epithelium • *Squamous* – *Keratinized* – *Non-keratinized* • *Columnar* • Cuboidal	 ***Skin, oral cavity, anus below white line*** ***Esophagus, anus up to white line, cornea and true vocal cords*** ***Salivary gland and conjunctiva*** ***Breast, sebaceous gland***
Pseudostratified columnar **Ciliated** **Non-ciliated**	 ***Respiratory epithelium, ductuli efferentes*** ***Vas deferens, seminal vesicle*** ***Membranous and penile urethra***

Transitional epithelium: Urothelium (BRUNN'S NEST- urothelium buried in the lamina propria of bladder)

Nerves

- Phrenic n C3, 4, 5
- Pudendal n S2, 3, 4
- Femoral/obturator n L2, 3, 4
- Sciatic n L4, 5 S1, 2, 3

Joints

Fibrous

- **Syndesmosis:**
  Inf tibiofibular jt

- **Cartilaginous:**
  Osteochondral, spheno-occipital

Synovial

- Ball and socket: Talocalcaneonavicular, incudostapedial, hip and shoulder jt
- Condylar: Knee, TMJ, atlanto-occipital
- Ellipsoid: Wrist, MCP
- Saddle: First carpometacarpal, sternoclavicular, calcaneocuboid, incudomalleolar
- Hinge: Elbow, ankle, interphalangeal
- Plane: Acromioclavicular, sternoclavicular, intercarpal, intertarsal
- Pivot: Inferior and superior radioulnar jt, atlantoaxial.

Foramen	Structure
F. Rotundum	Maxillary n
F. Spinosum	Middle meningeal artery
F. Ovale	Mandibular, accessory meningeal, lesser petrosal
F. Lacerum	Ascending pharyngeal
Jugular: Anterior Middle Posterior	 Inf. petrosal nerve 9, 10, 11 nerve IJV, occipital artery
Cranial nerves	**Efferents/afferents**
11	SVE
3, 4, 6, 12	GSE
3, 7, 9, 10	GVE
7, 9, 10	GVA
7, 9, 10	SVA
5	GSA
8	SSA

Surface Marking

Level	Structure
C 2 3	Oropharynx
C 4	Carotid bifurcation
C 6	Cricoids, chaisagne tubercle
T 4 5	Angle of lewis
T 7	Inf. angle of scapula
T 9	Xyphoid
T 12	Epiploic foramen
T 12 L 1	Coeliac artery
L 1	SMA, Suprarenal, Transpyloric plane, tip of 9th costal cartilage
L 1 2	Renal artery
Lower L1	Spinal cord end of adult
L2	Gonadal artery
L 3	IMA, Subcostal plane

Level	Structure
Lower L 3	Spinal cord end of infant
L 3 L 4	Umbilicus
Lower L 4	Iliac artery
Lower L 5	Iliac vein
S 2	Subarachnoid space, dura mater
S 4	Lower sigmoid mesocolon
C 1	Filum terminale

BLOOD SUPPLY OF HEART

RCA: Acute marginal artery
LCX: Obtuse marginal artery
LAD: Diagonal artery
Great cardiac vein: Anterior interventricular groove
Middle cardiac vein: Posterior interventricular groove.

Neuroanatomy (Concepts and facts)

- **GENERAL SOMATIC EFFERENT (GSE) NERVES:**
  - CN 3 (oculomotor), CN 4 (trochlear), CN 6 (abducens), CN 12 (hypoglossal)
- **GENERAL VISCERAL EFFERENT (GVE) NERVES:**
  - CN 3 (oculomotor), CN 7 (Facial nerve), CN 9 (Glossopharyngeal nerve), CN 10 (Vagus nerve)
- **SPECIAL VISCERAL EFFERENT (SVE) NERVES:**
  - *BRANCHIOMERIC NERVES (5, 7, 9, 10,* of branchial arch origin and *11)*
    - **Trigeminal nerve 5** innervates striated *muscle of mastication*
    - **Facial nerve 7** is the motor nerve for *muscles of facial expression*
    - **Glossopharyngeal nerve 9** innervates the *stylopharyngeus*
    - **Vagus nerve 10** innervates most of the *striated muscles of the larynx and pharynx.*
    - **Accessory nerve 11** is the motor nerve for the *sternocleidomastoid and trapezius.*
- **GENERAL VISCERAL AFFERENT (GVA) NERVES:**
  - CN 7 (Facial nerve), CN 9 (Glossopharyngeal nerve), CN 10 (Vagus nerve)
- **SPECIAL VISCERAL AFFERENT (SVA) NERVES:**
  - CN 7 (Facial nerve), CN 9 (Glossopharyngeal nerve), CN 10 (Vagus nerve)
- **GENERAL SOMATIC AFFERENT (GSA) NERVES:**
  - CN 5 (Trigeminal nerve).
- **SPECIAL SOMATIC AFFERENT (SSA) NERVES:**
  - CN 8 (Vestibulocochlear nerve).

Classification	Cranial nerves	Nuclei	Location
Motor			
Somatic Motor	III	Oculomotor nuclei	Ventral apex of the peri aqueductal gray of the mid brain at the superior colliculus
	IV	Trochlear nuclei	Ventral border of the peri aqeuductal gray, at the level of the inferior colliculus
	VI	Abducens nuclei	Caudal pons, beneath the floor of the 4th ventricle
	XII	Hypoglossal nuclei	Medulla

Classification	Cranial nerves	Nuclei	Location
Branchial Motor	V	Motor nucleus of trigeminal	Tegmentum of the mid pons
	VII	Facial nucleus	Caudal pontine tegmentum
	IX	Nucleus Ambiguus	Medulla
	X		
	XI	Accessory spinal nucleus	Caudal medulla
Parasympathetic	III	Edinger-Westphal nucleus	Midbrain peri aqueductal gray matter adjacent to the oculomotor nucleus
	VII	Superior salivary nucleus	Pontine tegmentum
	IX	Inferior salivary nucleus	Pontine tegmentum
	X	Dorsal motor nucleus	Medulla, Rostrally beneath the floor of the 4th ventricle lateral to the hypoglossal nucleus
Sensory			
Visceral special sensory	VII	Nucleus solitarius (rostral portion-gustatory nucleus)	Rostral medulla
	IX		
	X		
Visceral general sensory	IX	Nucleus solitarius (caudal portion-cardiorespiratory nucleus)	Caudal medulla
	X		
General somatic sensory	V	Trigeminal nuclei	Runs legnth of the brainstem into the cervical spinal cord
	VII		
	IX		
	X		
Special somatic sensory	VIII	Cochlear nuclei	Medulla near the lateral part of the floor of the fourth ventricle
		Vestibular nuclei	

- The pterion is superficial to the anterior branch of the middle meningeal artery, which supplies the dura and the skull.
- Pterion, the thinnest part of the calvaria → lateral skull fracture at the pterion → lacerate the middle meningeal artery → cause an epidural hematoma.
- Most of the meningeal dura is innervated by meningeal branches of the ophthalmic, maxillary, and mandibular divisions of the trigeminal nerve.
- The meningeal dura of the posterior cranial fossa is innervated by the first 3 cervical spinal nerves, and by the vagus n (CNX).
- Patients with a chronic subdural hematoma experience headache, impairment of cognitive skills, and gait instability.
- Primary olfactory neurons are continuously replaced. The life span of these cells ranges from 30 to 120 days in mammals.
- Hypoglossal nerve lesion causes deviation toward lesioned nerve on tongue on protrusion.
- Trochlear nerve is the only completely crossed cranial nerve and the only cranial nerve to arise from the dorsal aspect of the brain.
- Patients with a trochleor nerve lesion may tilt their head away from the side of the lesioned nerve; this results from a weakness in the ability to rotate the affected eyeball inward (intorsion). The head tilt is an attempt to counteract the extorsion by the unopposed inferior oblique and inferior rectus muscles.
- A head tilt observed in patients with a trochlear nerve lesion might be mistaken for torticollis that is caused by abnormal contractions of the sternocleidomastoid muscle.
- The abducens nerve is most commonly the first nerve to be affected in a thrombosis of the cavernous sinus.

CHAPTER 2

Embryology

Branchial Arches

Arches	Pouch	Mesoderm	Artery	Nerve
1	Tongue, ET tube, EAM is from cleft	Meckel's cartilage, mandible, malleus and incus, sphenomandibular ligament	–	Mandibular N
2	Tonsil	Stapes, styloid process, small horn and superior aspect of hyoid, richert's cartilage, stylohyoid ligament	Stapedial artery	Facial n
3	thymus, inf. parathyroid	Greater horn and inferior hyoid	Common carotid	Glossopharyngeal n
4	sup. parathyroid and thyroid	Laryngeal cartilage	Lt arch of aorta Rt subclavian	Sup. laryngeal
5	Ultimobranchial body, C cells	–	–	–
6		Arytenoids	Ductus arteriosus	Recurrent laryngeal nerve

Descent of Testis

Deep ring	6th month
Inguinal canal	7th month
Superficial ring	8th month
Scrotum	9th month

Aortic Arch

- Common carotid
- Left: Arch of aorta, Right: Subclavin artery
- Ductus venosus and pulm. artery
- Left subclavian artery.

1. Lt. common cardinal vein	CORONARY SINUS
2. Rt. Common cardinal vein	SVC
3. Rt. Vitelline vein	*TERMINAL* IVC
4. Septum primum	FOSSA OVALE
5. Septum secondum	LIMBUS FOSSA OVALE

HEART EMBRYOLOGY

Structure

- Truncus arteriosus (TA)
- Bulbus cordis

- Primitive ventricle
- Primitive atria
- Left horn of sinus venosus (SV)
- Right horn of SV
- Right common cardinal vein and right anterior cardinal vein

Derivative

- Ascending aorta and pulmonary trunk
- Right ventricle and smooth parts (outflow tract) of left and right ventricle
- Trabeculated left and right ventricles
- Trabeculated left and right atrium
- Coronary sinus
- Smooth part of right atrium
- SVC

← Dihydrotestosterone		Estrogen →
Glans penis	Genital tubercle	Glans clitoris
Corpus cavernosum and spongiosum	Genital tubercle	Vestibular bulbs
Bulbourethral glands (of Cowper)	Urogenital sinus	Greater vestibular glands (of Bartholin)
Prostate gland	Urogenital sinus	Urethral and paraurethral glands (of Skene)
Ventral shaft of penis (penile urethra)	Urogenital folds	Labia minora
Scrotum	Labioscrotal swelling	Labia majora

Concepts and Facts

- Primordial germ cells are from the epiblast from where they migrate to the yolk sac during the second week of development.
- In meiosis, in contrast to mitosis, however, **homologous chromosomes** then align themselves in **pairs,** a process called **synapsis.**
- The total number of germ cells is maximum by the fifth month of intrauterine life. It is around 7 million.
- Oocytes start forming by the third month of gestation.
- Oocytes are formed from oogonia when they enter meiosis 1. The meiosis is arrested in the prophase 1 in the diplotene stage. These cells are the primary oocytes.
- The primary oocytes can stay in the meiosis 1 even for 40 years or more until they are stimulated to complete their division.
- The primary oocytes carry 46 double structured chromosomes. (4n?)
- Primary oocyte plus the follicular cell is the primordial follicle.
- Just before ovulation the cell enters meiosis 2 but it is arrested in metaphase.
- The time required for a spermatogonium to become a mature spermatozoon is approximately 74 days.
- The theca interna cells produce androstenedione and testosterone while the granulosa cells convert it into estrone and 17-β estradiol.
- The LH surge at mid cycle causes the completion of meiosis 1 and initiation of meiosis 2 which gets arrested in the metaphase stage.
- Corpus luteum of pregnancy is called **corpus luteum graviditatis**.

- Binding and acrosome reaction are facilitated by a zona protein ZP3.
- In humans, both the head and the tail of the sperm enter the egg cytoplasm.
- The zona pellucida disappears by the 4th day after fertilization.
- New studies suggest that **L selectin** on trophoblast cells and its **carbohydrate receptors** on the uterine epithelium mediate initial attachment of the blastocyst to the uterus.
- Integrin receptors for laminin promote attachment, while those for fibronectin stimulate migration.
- Three distinct layers can be recognized in the endometrium in the secretory phase: a superficial **compact layer**, an intermediate **spongy layer**, and a thin **basal layer.**
- Fusion begins in the cervical region (fifth somite) and proceeds cranially and caudally.
- Closure of the cranial neuropore occurs at approximately day 25 (18- to 20-somite stage), whereas the posterior neuropore closes at day 28 (25-somite stage)
- Insulin like growth factor-2 is highly expressed in capillary hemangioma.
- Each nucleosome consists of an octamer of histone proteins and approximately 140 base pairs of DNA.
- WT1 gene (Wilm's tumor) shows splice variants. For example, isoforms of the WT1 gene have different functions in gonadal versus kidney development.
- Notch signalling is especially important in neuronal differentiation, blood vessel specification, and somite segmentation.
- FGF8 is important for development of the limbs and parts of the brain.

CHAPTER 3

Histology

- Reticular fibers consist mainly of collagen type III.
- The elastic fiber system is composed of three types of fibers—oxytalan, elaunin, and elastic.
- Microfibrils composed of various glycoproteins, including **fibromodulin I and II** and a large molecule called **fibrillin.**
- Mutations in the fibrillin gene result in Marfan syndrome, a disease characterized by a lack of resistance in the tissues rich in elastic fibers. Large arteries → rich in components of the elastic system → blood pressure is high in the aorta → patients with this disease often experience aortic rupture.
- Elastic tissue, which occurs infrequently, is present in the yellow ligaments of the vertebral column and in the suspensory ligament of the penis.
- Mucous tissue has an abundance of ground substance composed primarily of hyaluronic acid. It is a jellylike tissue containing very few fibers. The cells in this tissue are mainly fibroblasts. Mucous tissue is the principal component of the umbilical cord, where it is referred to as **Wharton's jelly.** It is also found in the pulp of young teeth.
- Collagen, hyaluronic acid, proteoglycans, and small amounts of several glycoproteins are the principal macromolecules present in all types of cartilage matrix. Elastic cartilage, characterized by its great pliability, contains significant amounts of the protein elastin in the matrix.
- As a consequence of various functional requirements, three forms of cartilage have evolved, each exhibiting variations in matrix composition.
- In the matrix of **hyaline cartilage,** the most common form, type II collagen is the principal collagen type the more pliable and distensible **elastic cartilage** possesses, in addition to collagen type II, an abundance of elastic fibers within its matrix.
- **Fibrocartilage,** present in regions of the body subjected to pulling forces, is characterized by a matrix containing a dense network of coarse type I collagen fibers.
- In adult mammals, hyaline cartilage is located in the articular surfaces of the movable joints, in the walls of larger respiratory passages (nose, larynx, trachea, bronchi), in the ventral ends of ribs, where they articulate with the sternum, and in the **epiphyseal plate,** where it is responsible for the longitudinal growth of bone.
- Cartilage proteoglycans contain chondroitin 4-sulfate, chondroitin 6-sulfate, and keratan sulfate, covalently linked to core proteins. Up to 200 of these proteoglycans are noncovalently associated with long molecules of hyaluronic acid, forming **proteoglycan aggregates** that interact with collagen. The aggregates can be up to 4 m in length.
- In addition to type II collagen and proteoglycan, an important component of cartilage matrix is the structural glycoprotein **chondronectin,** a macromolecule that binds specifically to glycosaminoglycans and collagen type II, mediating the adherence of chondrocytes to the extracellular matrix. The cartilage matrix surrounding each chondrocyte is rich in glycosaminoglycan and poor in collagen. This peripheral zone, called the **territorial,** or **capsular,** matrix, stains differently from the rest of the matrix.
- Elastic cartilage is found in the auricle of the ear, the walls of the external auditory canals, the auditory (eustachian) tubes, the epiglottis, and the cuneiform cartilage in the larynx.
- In areas of bone undergoing resorption, osteoclasts lie within enzymatically etched depressions in the matrix known as **Howship's lacunae.**

- α-Actinin and desmin (an intermediate filament protein) are believed to tie adjacent sarcomeres together, thus keeping the myofibrils in register.
- Lipofuscin pigment granules (aging pigment), often seen in long-lived cells, are found near the nuclear poles of cardiac muscle cells.
- **Desmin (skeletin)** has been identified as the major protein of intermediate filaments in all smooth muscles, and **vimentin** is an additional component in vascular smooth muscle.
- In addition to contractile activity, smooth muscle cells also synthesize collagen, elastin, and proteoglycans, which are extracellular products normally associated with the function of fibroblasts.
- Smooth muscle is capable of an active regenerative response. After injury, viable mononucleated smooth muscle cells and pericytes from blood vessels undergo mitosis and provide for the replacement of the damaged tissue.
- The internal surface of all components of the blood and lymphatic systems is lined by a single layer of a squamous epithelium, called endothelium.

CHAPTER 4

Physiology

- Forebrain (Procencephalon) – Telencephalon (lat. ventricle) + Diencephalon (3rd ventricle, thalamus, hypothalamus, metathalamus, epithalamus, subthalamus)
- Midbrain (Mesencephalon) – Midbrain Aqueduct, tectum, tegmentum
- Hindbrain (Rhomboncephalon) Metencephalon (pons and cerebellum) Myencephalon (medulla and spinal cord)
- Rhinencephalon – smell
- Corpus striatum = caudate nucleus + lentiform nucleus (globus pallidum and putamen)
- Striatum = Caudate nucles and putamen

Cerebellum	Structure	Function
Archicerebellum	Vestibulocerebellum (floculonodular)	Balance, axial muscles
Paleocerebellum	Spinocerebellum (Fastigial, globose)	Execution, posture, tone, coordination
Neocerebellum	Dendate nucleus	Planning and programming

Merocrine	Simple sweat gland, pancreas, protein by mammay gland
Apocrine	Sweat, fat by mammary
Holocrine	Sebaceous gland

Bohr effect	Decrease in oxygen affinity when pH falls and pCO_2 increases.
Haldane effect	Binding of oxygen decreases affinity for CO_2 (ISohydric transport of CO_2)
Hamberger effect	Chloride shift

Shift of Curve to Left

- Increased pH
- Decreased temp
- CO Hb
- Fetal Hb
- Decreased pCO_2
- Decreased 2, 3 DPG
- Meth Hb
- Stored blood

Shift to Right

- Decreased pH
- Increased temperature
- High altitude
- Anemia
- Increased CO_2
- Increased 2, 3 DPG
- Sickle Hb
- Exercise

TRANSPORTERS

GLUT 1	Placenta brain RBC kidney
GLUT 2	Beta cell kidney small intestine liver (insulin independent)
GLUT 3	Brain, placenta, kidney
GLUT 4	Skeletal muscle, cardiac muscle, adipose tissue (insulin dependant)
GLUT 5	Jejunum sperm (fructose)
GLUT 6	–
SGLT 1	Small intestine, renal tubule 2 Na
SGLT 2	Renal tubule 1 Na
GLUT 7	Transport in ER-liver

Smoking Protects Against

- PIH
- Fibroid
- Endometriosis
- CA Endometrium
- Ulcerative colitis
- Alzheimer's disease

Progesterone: Increased basal body temperature, Increased weight, insulin resistance

C 18	Estrogen
C 19	Testosterone/androgen
C 21	Progesterone/cortisol

EPSP and IPSP

Fast EPSP	ACh nicotinic
Slow EPSP	ACh M 2 decreased potassium conductance
Late slow EPSP	GnRH
Slow IPSP	Dopamine, increased potassium conductance

Receptor	Sensation
Free nerve ending	Pain
Meissner's corpuscle	Tapping
Pacinian corpuscle	Trickle, vibration
Merkel's disc	Pressure
Krausse end bulb	Cold
Ruffini's end organ	Touch, pressure

Erlanger-Gasser Classification

A Alpha	Proprioception, somatic motor
A Beta	Touch, pressure, motor
A Gamma	Muscle spindle, motor
A Delta	Fast pain, cold, touch
B	Preganglionic autonomic
C	Slow pain, sympathetic postganglionic

Hypoxia = B > A > C
Pressure = A > B > C
Local anesthesia = C > B > A
Golgi tendon organ: *Inverse stretch type*
Golgi **bottle** neuron: *Reciprocal innervations*
Adaptation: Decreased response with *constant stimulus*
Accomodation: Increased threshold with *subthreshold stimulus*

Hypothalamus

Suprachiasmatic	Diurnal variation
Arcuate nucleus	GnRH, prolactin
Supraoptic	Vasopressin
Preoptic	Thirst
Anterior hypothalamus	Osmoreceptor
Lateral hypothalamus	Thirst and hunger
Paraventricular	Oxytocin
Ventromedial	Satiety
Lateral hypothalamus	Hunger and thirst
Nucleus accumbens, medial forebrain bundle	Reward

Plasma osmolality–290 mosmol/lit
GFR-125 ml/min or 180 l/day
Urine acidity-4.5
Actual RPF-700 ml/min
Effective RPF-625 ml/min

Osmolarity of Tubular Fluid

DCT	Hypotonic
PCT, CT	Isotonic
TDL	Hypertonic
AL	Hypertonic

Types of Bladder

Atonic bladder	Deafferentation, *e.g. tabes dorsalis*
Automatic bladder	Denervation
Autonomic bladder	Spinal cord mediated, cortical control lost

Countercurrent *multiplier:* Henle's loop
Contercurrent *exchanger:* Vasarecta

GASTRIN: Increased by vagus, calcium, adrenalline, GRP, trypsin and pancreatic amylase. Decreased by acid, stomatostain, secretin, GIP, VIP, glucogon and calcitonin. ↑Gastric juice ↑Gastric motility ↑Insulin after protein meal	**GIP:** K cells ↓Gastric secretion ↓Gastric motility ↑Insulin

Contd...

Contd...

CHOLECYSTOKININ (CCK):	**VASO INTESTINAL POLYPEPTIDE (VIP):**
More enzyme, less volume ↓Gastric emptying ↓Gall bladder motility ↓Small intestine motility ↓Pyloric spasm	↑Increased electrolyte secretion ↓Gastric secretion Relaxation of all smooth muscles
SECRETIN: Watery alkaline juice ↑HCO_3 ↓Gastrin ↓Gastric acid ↓Gastric motility	**STOMATOSTATIN:** Decreases all secretions

PANCREATIC CELLS

α – Glucagon
β – Insulin
δ – Stomatostatin
F – Pancreatic polypeptide
D1 – VIP
G – Gastrin
K – GIP

RESPIRATORY BURST

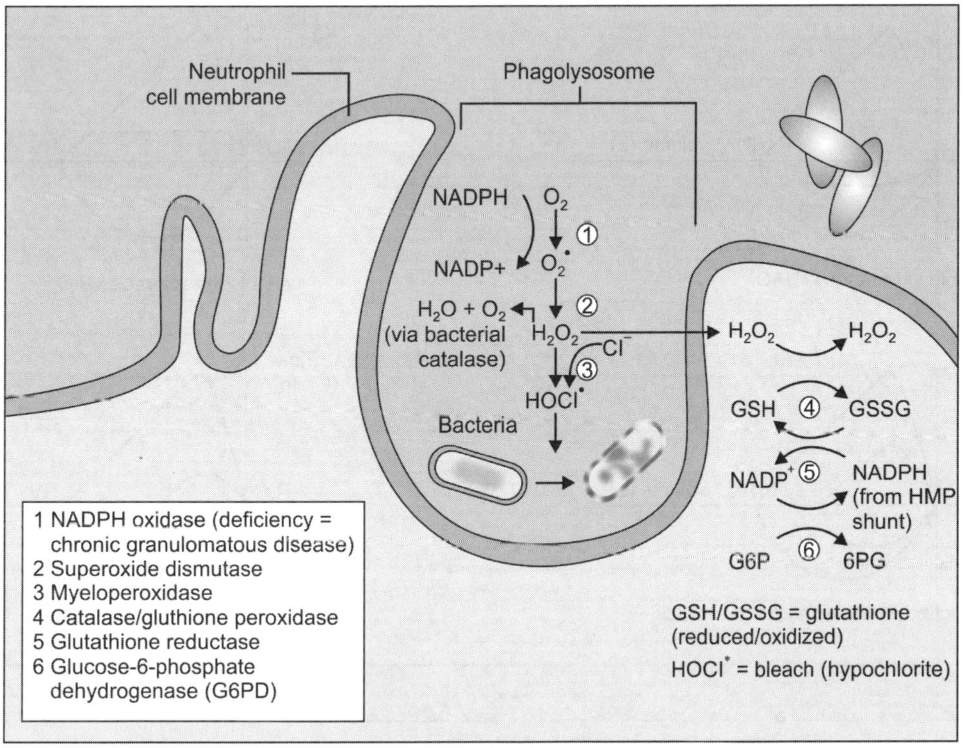

Fig. 4.1: Respiratory burst

Applied Pulmonary Physiology: (Blue-Normal, Maroon-Described Condition)

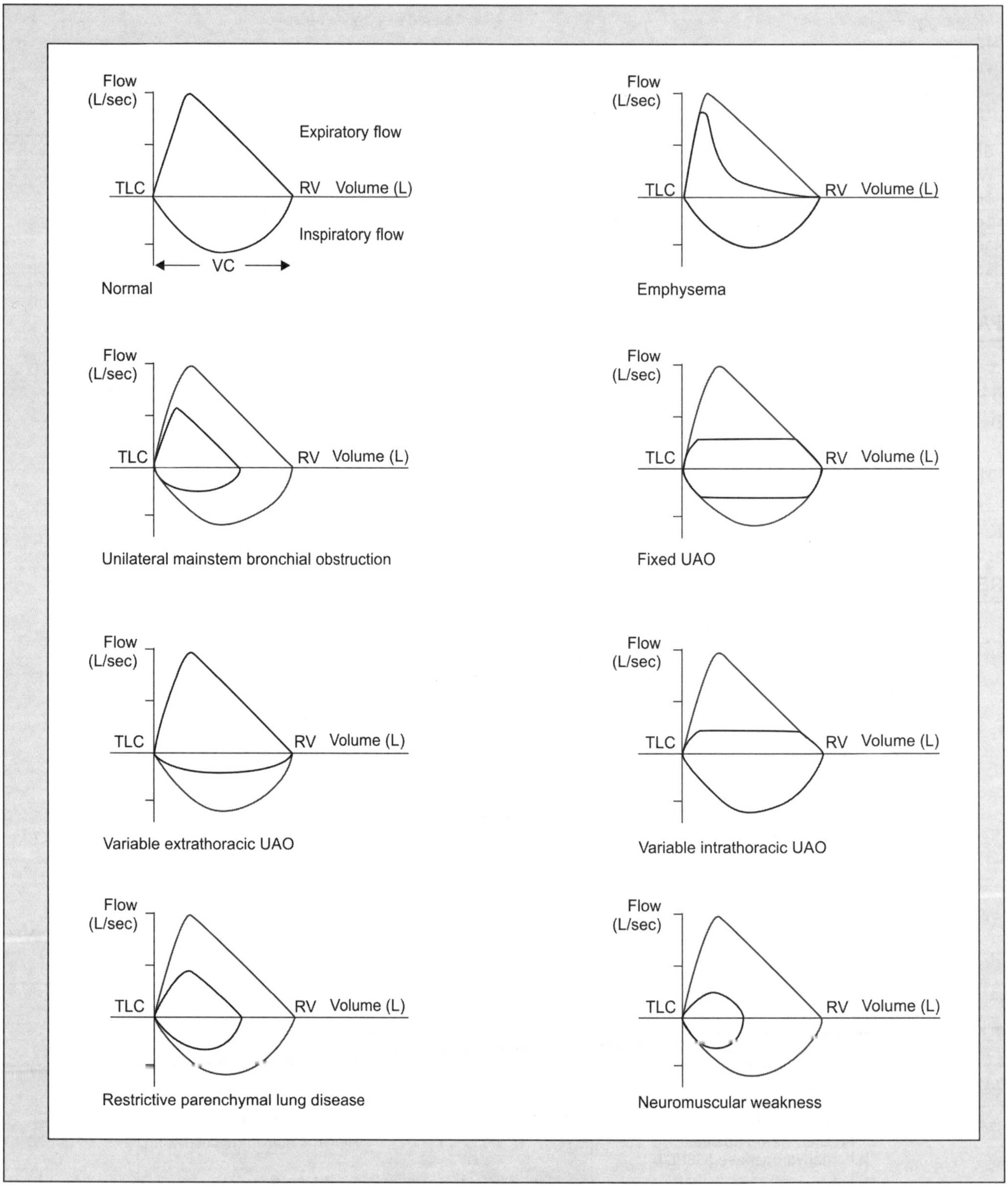

Fig. 4.2: Spirometry

- Hamburger effect—Chloride shift-CO_2 produced in tissues-enters RBCs-Carbonic Anhydrase-CO_2 combines with H_2O-forms $H_2CO_3^-$ splits into H^+ and HCO_3^- ions-HCO_3^- exchanged for Cl via Band 3-Cl-enters RBCs in capillaries-hence venous blood shows lower Cl-conc and higher hematocrit
- 1, 3 BPG—converted by BPG Mutase to-2, 3BPG-allosteric effector-binds with greater affinity to deoxygenated hemoglobin—decreasing their affinity for oxygen-allosterically promotes the release of the remaining oxygen molecules bound to the hemoglobin—Fetal Hb shows low affinity for 23 BPG—binds tightly to O_2
- Countercurrent multiplier—consists of two parallel limbs of renal tubules running in opposite directions—descending limb of the loop of Henle is permeable to water but impermeable to solutes—making the filtrate hypertonic—ascending limb is impermeable to water but permeable to solutes—Na^+, Cl^-, and K^+ are actively transported into the medullary space, making the filtrate hypotonic— multiplication process—the countercurrent flow within the descending and ascending limb increases, or *multiplies* the osmotic gradient between tubular fluid and interstitial space.
- Na K ATPase pump—pumps 3 Na ions out and 2 K ions-creates net negative charge inside the cell
- Gq type G protein—activates PLC-hydrolyses PIP2 to IP3 and DAG-former opens up Ca channels and latter activates protein kinase C.

CHAPTER 5

Biochemistry

RATE-LIMITING ENZYME

Urea cycle	Carbomyl PO_4 synthetase-p-mito
Cholestoral synthesis	HMG CoA reductase
Ketone synthesis	HMG CoA synthetase
Fatty acid synthesis ACC	Acetyl CoA Carboxylase
HMP Pathway	G6PD
Haeme synthesis	ALA synthase
Bile acid synthesis	7 OH lase
Catecholamine synthesis	Tyrosine OH lase
Melanin synthesis	Tyrosinase
Glycolysis	Phosphofructokinase (PFK)
Translation	IF -4E binding to cap
Purine synthesis	Phosphoribosyl amino transferase
Pyrimidine synthesis	Aspartate Transcarbamalyase -ATC
Kreb cycle	Iso citrate dehydrogenase
Gluconeogenesis	Pyruvate carboxylase PEPCK
Uric acid synthesis	Xanthine oxidase

BLOTTING TECHNIQUES

- Northern blot—RNA
- Southern blot—DNA
- Western blot—Protein
- Southwestern blot—DNA-binding protein

Amino acids

Nonpolar

- Alanine
- Leucine
- Methionine
- Phenylalanine
- Valine
- Isoleucine
- Proline
- Tryptophan

Nonionic Polar

- Glycine
- Threonine
- Tyrosine
- Asparagine
- Serine
- Cysteine
- Glutamine

Acidic

- Aspartic acid
- Glutamic acid

Basic (BHAL)

- Histidine
- Arginine
- Lysine

Ketogenic

- Lysine
- Isoleucine
- Tyrosin
- Leucine
- Phenylalanine
- Tryptophan

Dibasic Monocarboxylic

- Arginine
- Lysine

Ionic Polar

Amino acids	Functional group
Methionine	Thioether
Arginine	Guanidium
Histidine	Imidazole
Tryptophan	Indolo
Proline	Pyrolidine

Essential Amino acids

TTV HILL MAP no GAPS

- Threonine
- Valine
- Isoleucine
- Lysine
- Arginine
- Tryptophan
- Histidine
- Leucine
- Methionine
- Phenylalanine

Partially Essential

- Histidine
- Arginine

Markers

Plasma membrane	Adenyl cyclase 5 nucleotidase Na K ATPase
Cytoplasm	LDH
ER microsome	Glucose 6 phospatase
Lysosome	ATP, Cathepsin
Golgi app	Galactosyl transferase
Mitochondria	Glutamate dehydrogenase
Peroxisome	Catalase Uric acid oxidase

Enzymes

Oxidoreductase	Aldehyde dehydrogenase, tyrosinase
Transferase	Hexokinase, phosporylase, phosphomutokinase
Hydrolase	ACH esterase, trypsi, lipase, urease, ALP, pepsin
Lyases	Aldolase
Isomerase	Fumarase, histidase
Ligase	Acetyl CoA carboxylase, PRPP synthetase

LDH-1	H_4	Heart
2	$H_3 M_1$	RBC
3	$H_2 M_2$	Brain
4	$H_1 M_3$	Liver
5	M_4	Muscle

Ketogenic AA

Acetyl CoA, valine, isoleucine, methionine—Succinyl CoA, Arginine, histidine, proline, Alpha Ketoglutarate, alanine, cystine, serine, glycine, threonine-pyruvate.

RNA POLYMERASE

Start-sigma
Stop-Rho

I A	rRNA
II B	mRNA
III C	sRNA
Prokaryotes	2 alpha, 1 beta

DNA POLYMERASE

I	α	Gapfilling in lagging strand
II	£	Proofreading
II	β	DNA repair
II	γ	Mito DNA
III	Δ	Leading strand

GAG TYPES

Hyaluronic acid	Synovial fluid, cartilage, vitreous humor, loose connective tissue
Chondroitin sulfate	Cornea, cartilage bone
Keratin sulfate	Cornea KSI, loose connective tissues
Heparin sulfate	Aortic wall, skin fibroblast
Dermatan sulfate	Pliability of skin valves, cornea

Hyaluronic acid	D glucoronic acid+ n acetyl glucosamine
Chondroitin sulfate	D glucoronic acid+ n acetyl galactosamine 4 sulfate
Heparin	D glucoronate 2 sulfate+ N sulfoglucosamine 6 sulfate
Dermatan sulfate	L iduronic acid+ N acetyl galactosamine 4 sulfate
Keratan sulfate	D galactose+ N acetylglucosamine 6 sulfate

VITAMINS AND COENZYMES

Thiamine (TPP) Oxidecarboxylation

- Pyruvate dehydrogenase
- Transketolase
- Alpha ketoglutarate dehydrogenase
- Branched chain ketoacids

Pyridoxine B_6

- Glycogen phosporylase
- Glycine cleavage system
- Decarboxylase
- Kinurinase
- Tranaminase
- Cystatheine synthetase

Biotin

- Proponyl CoA carboxylase
- Acetyl CoA carboxylase

Pantothenic Acid

- Acyl carrier protein
- Acetylation

Vitamin B_{12}

- Leucine aminomutase
- Methionine synthetase
- Ribonucleotide
- Propionyl CoA mutase
- Ethylene glycol

Fatty Acid Oxidation ATP

[n-2] × 5/2 + **(n/2) × 12**

Italicized—from beta oxidation, bold—from TCA

Disease	Enzyme deficiency
Amino acids	
Tyrosinemia I	Fumarylacetoacetate hydroxylase
Tyrosinemia II or Richner Hanhart Syndrome	Tyrosine aminotransferase
Alkaptonuria	Homogentisate oxidase
Phenylketonuria	Phenylalanine OH-lase
MSUD	Alpha keto acid decarboxylase

Disease	Enzyme deficiency
Hartnup	Neutral AA transporter
Cystinuria	Cystine, ornithine, lysine, arginine excretion in urine
Cystathionuria	Cystathionase
Homocystinuria	Cystathione beta synthase
Primary oxaluria	Alanine glyoxylate aminotransferase
Glycogen storage disease (I–VII)	
von Gierke's	G-6-PO4ase
Pompe	Acid maltase
Cori/Forbes	Debranching
Anderson	Branching
McArdle's	Muscle PO4ase
Her's	Liver PO4ase
Tauri	PFK
Other carbohydrates	
Essential fructosuria	Fructokinase
Hereditary fructose intolerance	Aldolase B
Galactosemia	Gal-1-PO4 uridyl transferase, UDP-Gal epimerase, Galactokinase
Essential pentosuria	Xylitol DHase
Lysosomal storage diseases	
Tay-Sachs	Hexosaminidase A
Sandhoff	Hexosaminidase A and B
Fabry's	Alpha Galactosidase
Krabbe's	Beta Galactosidase
Gaucher	Alpha glucosidase
Neimann Pick	Sphingomyelinase
Farber's	Ceramidase
Mucopolysaccharidosis	
Hurler	Iduronidase
Hunter	Iduronate sulfatase
San-Fillipo	Multiple enzymes involved, Heparan SO4 accumulation
Morquio	
Maroteaux-Lamy	Arylsulfatase B
Sly	Beta glucuronidase
Urea cycle defects	
Hyperammonemia I	CPS-1
Hyperammonemia II	Ornithine transcarbomylase
Citrullinemia	Arginosuccinate synthase
Arginosuccinic aciduria	Argininosuccinase deficiency
Gyrate atrophy	Ornithine aminotransferase
Purine/Pyrimidines	
Lesch Nyhan	HGPRTase
SCID	Adenosine deaminase
Orotic aciduria I	Orotate phosphoribosyl transferase + Orotidylate decarboxylase

Disease	Enzyme deficiency
Orotic aciduria II	Orotidylate decarboxylase
Miscellaneous	
Adreno leukodystrophy (ALD)	VLCFA oxidation defect in peroxisome
Refsum	Alpha phytanic acid oxidase
Canavan	Aspartoacylase deficiency

Molecule	Composition
Sphingomyelin	Sphingosine + Choline
Sialic acid	NANA-Ganglioside
Lecithin	Phosphatidylcholine
Cephalin	Phosphatidyl ethanolamine
Cardiolipin	Diphosphatidyl glycerol
Ceramide	Sphingosine + FA

Saturated Fatty Acids

Source	Fatty acid
Butter (BBC)	Butyric acid (4) Caproic acid (6)
Coconut (CLM)	Lauric acid (12) Myristic acid (14)
Body stores	Palmitic acid (16) Stearic acid (18)

Biochemical Tests

Carbohydrate	Test
Reducing sugar	Benedict's, Fehling
Monosaccharide	Barfoed
Fructose	Seliwanoff and Foulger's
5C sugars	Molish

Test	Biochemical mechanism and AA
Heller	Ninhydrin formation
Biuret	2 peptide bonds
Millon	Phenol groups (not phenlyalanine)
Xanthoprotein	Benzene ring AA
Aldehyde	Tryptophan
Sakaguchi	Arginine (Guanidium group)
Nitroprusside	SH group (Homocysteine)
Pauling	Tyrosine

Tests for bile pigments:

- Fouchet's
- Van der Bergh
- Gmelin
- Ehrlich and Schelsinger (urobilinogen)

Tests for bile salts:

- *Pettenkoffer*
- *Hay's*

Tests for ketones:

- Gerhardt's
- Rothera's

Tests for disease

Guthrie	PKU
$FeCl_3$	PKU and Alkaptonuria
Nitrosonaphthol	Tyrosinemia
Bail	Essential pentosuria
DNPH	MSUD
Obermeyer	Hartnup
Mucic Acid	Galactosuria

Steroid Synthesis

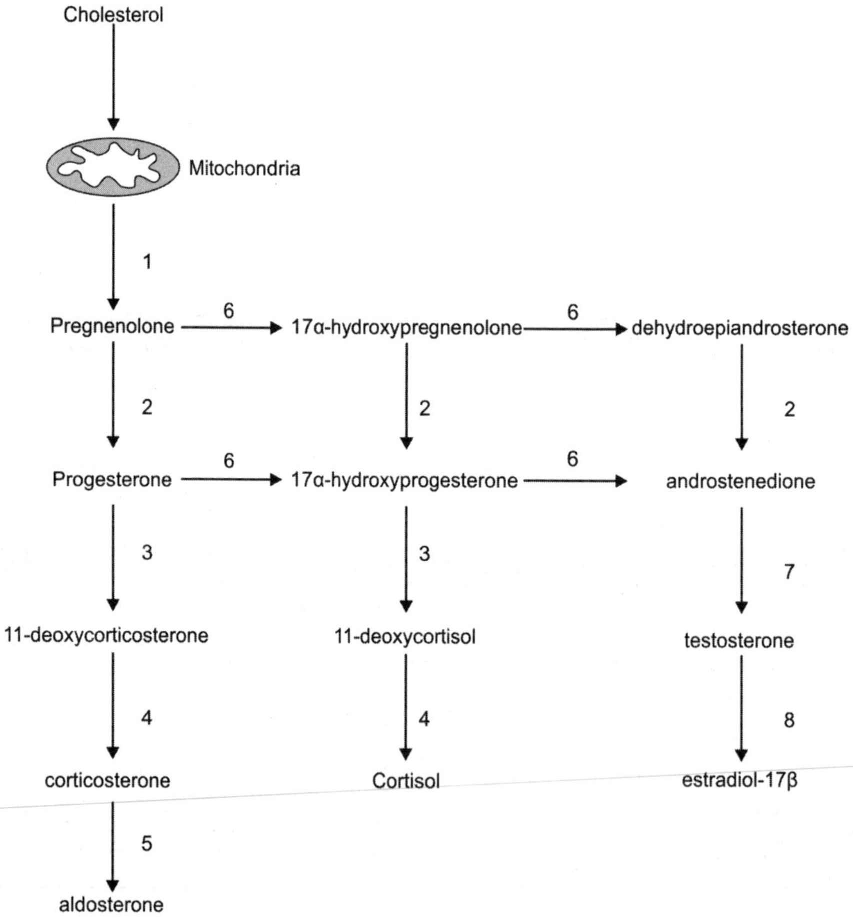

(1) Cytochrome P450 side chain cleavage; (2) 3β-hydroxysteroid dehydrogenase/Δ5–Δ4 isomerase; (3) Cytochrome P450 21-hydroxylase; (4) Cytochrome P450 11β-hydroxylase; (5) Aldosterone synthase; (6) Cytochrome P450 17α-hyroxylase/C17-20 lyase; (7) 17β-hydroxysteroid dehydrogenase; (8) Cytochrome P450 aromatase.

Easy way to remember defects in Congenital Adrenal Hyperplasia:

- Firstly, just remember the numbers **11, 17 and 21**
- When there is **1 in the ten's place** (e g. 11 or 17) then there will be **hypertension**
- When there is **1 in the unit's place** (e g. 11 or 21) there is **virilization**
- In **11-beta-OHlase** deficiency there is **both hypertension and virilization.**

Hemoglobin	Globin Chains
A	α2, β2
A2	α2, δ2
F	α2, γ2
H	β4
Bart	γ4
S	Valine
C	Lysine
D	Glutamate—Glutamine

Peroxisomal Enzymes

- Uric acid oxidation
- D-amino acid oxidase
- Catalase
- Fatty acid oxidation

NEONATAL HYPOGLYCEMIA CAUSES

- Glycogen storage disorder – type 1
- Fructose intolerance
- Galactosemia
- Medium chain fatty acyl CoA dehydrogenase deficiency
- Long chain fatty acyl CoA dehydrogenase deficiency

ENZYMES THAT CONTAIN ZINC

- Superoxide dismutase
- Carbonic anhydrase
- Aldehyde dehydrogenase
- ALA dehydratase
- Alkaline phosphatase
- LDH
- Glutamate dehydrogenase
- DNA and RNA polymerase

TCA

- Amphibolic cycle: both oxidative and synthetic
- Anaplerotic reaction: Filling 'up', "in or out"
- 4 'c' are used continuously (heme synt succ CoA)
- To fill up these TCA works.

Toxins Acting on TCA Cycle

Fluoroacetate × aconitase

Arsenite × Alpha-ketoglutarate dehydrogenase (α-KGDH)

Arsenite × phosphoglycerate kinase ←
Fluoride × Enolase ← → Irreversible

Iodoacetate × Glyceraldehyde-3-phosphate dehydrogenase (GAPD)

Arsenite ×
Mercury × → Pyruvate dehydrogenase (PDH complex)

Malonate ×
Oxaloacetate × → succinate dehydrogenase

Hypoglycin × Free Fatty Oxidation (Jamaican vomiting sickness – ripe fruit of Ackee tree)

Malate-aspartate Shuttle

Oxaloacetic acid (OAA) important to mitochondria, so NADPH produced in glycolysis is transferred through malate.

Gly-3-PO_4/DHAP shuttle (glycerol-3-phosphate/Dihydroxyacetone phosphate shuttle)

Brain and muscle only

FAD—2 ATP

PASTEUR EFFECT × CRABTREE EFFECT

Pasteur effect:

- Aerobic oxidation inhibits anerobic degradation of glucose
- O_2 inhibits glycolysis
- Decreased O_2 increases glycolysis

Crabtree effect:

- Constant O_2 supply—increased glucose—increased anaerobic glycolysis

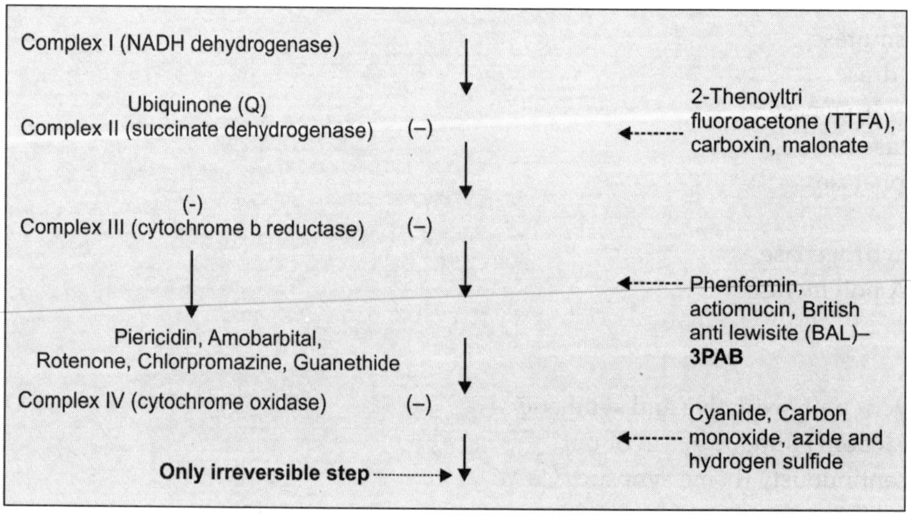

Mitochondrial myopathy, encephalopathy, lactic acidosis, and stroke (MELAS) – I and IV deficiency

ATP synthase:

F1 inside
3 α
3 β 9PP
1 γ - axel
1 σ
1 ε

Uncouplers:

- 2–4 dinitrophenol
- 2–4 dinitrocresol
- CCCP (Chlorocarbonylcyanidephenyl hydrazone)

Physiological Uncouplers:

- Thyroxine
- Long chain fatty acid in Brown tissue
- Unconjugated bilirubin

Inhibition of Oxidative Phosphorylation:

- Atractyloside × ADP-ATP translocase
- Oligomycin × inhibits flow of protons through F_o
- Valinomycin × Iodophores
- Gramicidin, a channel-forming peptide on membrane
- Phosphofructokinase 2 (PFK2): Fructose 2, 6 bisphosphatase – inhibits Gluconeogenesis
- Tandem Effect
- Bifunctional
- Anti-phosphofructokinase 1 (PFK1) – inhibits Fructose 1, 6 bisphosphatase

Pentosuria:

- Benedicts test: +ve
- Bials test: +ve

Transamination:

- Pyruvate ↔ Alanine
- Oxaloacetate ↔ Aspartate
- α – keto glutarate ↔ Glutamate

Substrate Level Phosphorylation: 3 Kinase

- Pyruvate kinase
- Succinyl thiokinase – TCA
- Phosphoglycerate kinase

Glycolysis	**Gluconeogenesis** (corresponding step)
Hexokinase	Glucose 6 phosphatase
Phosphofructokinase (PFK)	Fru 1, 6 bisphosphatase
Pyruvate kinase	Phosphoenolpyruvate carboxykinase (PEPCK) (GTP) ← Succinate dehydrogenase
Pyruvate dehydrogenase (PDH)	Pyruvate carboxylase
Phosphoglycerate kinase generates ATP	If catalyzed by Phosphoglycerate kinase, reaction proceeds in opposite direction, generates ADP and 1, 3-BPG

Anomer: α_1 β 1st carbon 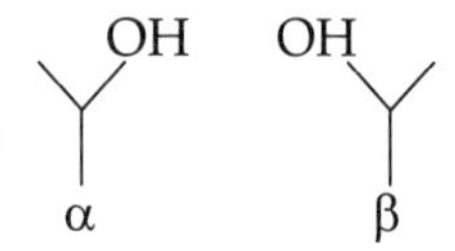

Epimer:
1st and Penultimate in glucose
2nd Mannose and 4th -Galactose

Enantiomer: D, L mirror image with Penultimate carbon

Optical activity: d (+), l (–)

Diastereomer – no mirror image but similar structure
Sucrose: Glu-Fru α 1 → 2
Inulin: Fru-Fru β 1 → 2
Cellulose: Glu-Glu β 1 → 4
Lactose: Gal-Glu β1 → 4
Maltose: Glu-Glu α 1 → 4
Isomerase: Glu-Glu α 1 → 6
Starch: Glu-Glu α 1 → 4
Enediol: HO–C=C–OH
For free aldo/keto group

Molisch test: Furfural
Need 5 carbon
H_2SO_4
Osazone formation with Phenyl hydrazine
Glu-Fru-Mannose → Needle shaped
Lactose → Hedgehog
Maltose → Sunflower

Benedict's Test

$CuSO_4$
Na_2CO_3
Sodium citrate
$Cu^{2+} \rightarrow Cu^{1+}$(cuprous)
Not for Non reducing sugars: Starch, Sucrose, Trehalose.

Oxidation

- Ald: Gluconic acid
- Keto: Glucoronic acid
- First carbon: Aldonic acid
- Last carbon: Uronic acid
- Both: Saccharic acid

Reduction

- Aldehyde → Alcohol
- D-glucose → Sorbitol
- D-fructose → Sorbitol and mannitol
- Galactose → Dulcitol

Hydrolysis of Starch

Starch (NR) – Blue
↓
Amylodextrin (NR) – Violet
↓
Erythrodextrin (mild R) – Red
↓
Achrodextrin (R) – No color

R-Reducing/NR-non reducing

β-D Glycanopyranose – Common
α-D Glucopyranose – Crystalline glucose

Amylase $\alpha\ 1 \rightarrow 4$
↓

α	β (dextrinogenic)
random	from end stop at $\alpha\ 1 \rightarrow 6$ (branch)
↓	↓
α – maltose	large limit dextrins

STARCH
↓

Amylose 20%	Amylopectin 80%
↓	↓
Non branching	Branching
$\alpha\ 1 \rightarrow 4$	$\alpha\ 1 \rightarrow 6$

L- Fucose – deoxygalactose

H–C=O H- C_2–OH HO- C_3–H H- C_4–OH H- C_5–OH CH_2OH D–Glucose Open projection formular	OH H-1C H-2C-OH O HO-$_3$C-H H-4C-OH H-5C 6CH_2OH α-D–Glucose Closed ring structure Fischer formular (Hemiacetal)
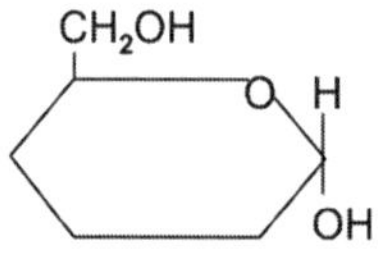 α-D–Glucopyranose Howarth formula	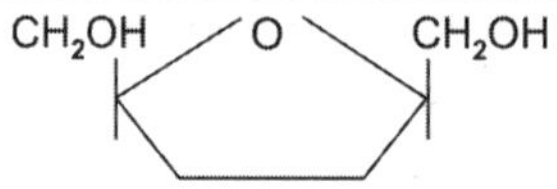 α-D–Fructo furanose Howarth formula

3×10^9 Base pairs in DNA - Haploid

RNA	DNA (alk. Resi)
Adenine	Adenine
Guanine	Guanine
Cytosine	Cytosine
Uracil	*Thymine*

ssRNA – Small stable – Regulation

snRNA – Small nucleus – RNA processing

mRNA – 5′ ———————— 3′

CH_3GTP capping   Poly 'A' tail

tRNA –

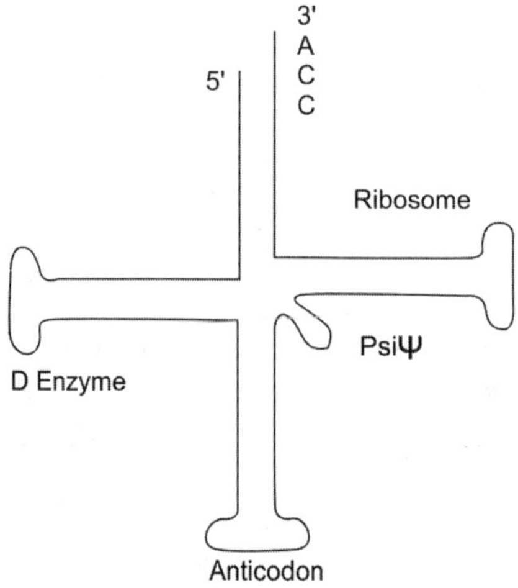

Acceptable missense	Hb Hikari
Partially acceptable missense	Hb S
Unacceptable missense	Hb M (Boston) ~ bad

Silent Mutation	
Hbi Milwaukee	Glutamate
Bristol	Aspartate
Sydney	Alanine

Telomerase → TTAGGG 5' 3'

A + G = T + C   A + G/T + C ~ 1

AAA	Lysine
GGG	Glycine
CCC	Proline
UUU (TTT)	Phenylalanine

Peptidyl transfer – 28S of 60S ribounit of rRNA

A ≡ T

C ≡ G

rRNA

Eukaryotic – 60 S + 40 S = 80 S

Prokaryotic – 50 S + 30 S = 70 S

Double Helix – DNA:

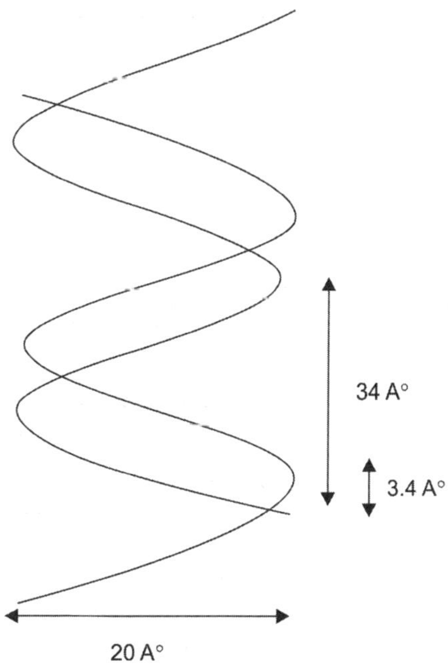

61 + 3	Codon
Coding strand	5' → 3'
Template strand	3' → 5'
m-RNA	5' → 3'

31	t-RNA (22 mitochondrial)
20	AA

START – AUG – Methionine

STOP – UAA, UAG, UGA
(Ochre, Amber, Opal)
Non sense mutation

TRANSLATION:

Kozak sequence - Eukaryotes *(rho absent in eukaryotes)

Shine Dalgarno sequence - Prokaryotes *(sigma start)
Near AUG

Transcription	
TATA box TATAAT	Prokaryotes (Pribnow box – bacteria)
Goldberg hogness TATAAAAG	Eukaryotes

IF 1–3 → Pre initiation complex	
IF 4E → Cap binding (rate limiting)	
IF 4B → ATPase	4 2 ATP 2 GTP
IF 5 → GTPase	
Diptheria toxin → inhibits elongation factor: eEF_2	

Klenow Fragment is an N-terminal truncation of DNA Polymerase I which retains polymerase activity, but has lost the 5′ → 3′ exonuclease activity

Topoisomerases I	Topoisomerases II
Relaxes super coil	Transient block Relaxes both positive and negative supercoils Can insert supercoiling
Topotecans: Inhibitor of topoisomerase I	ATP gyrase Introduce negative supercoil Gyrase A Gyrase B Nalidixic acid Novobiocin • Podophyllotoxin • Anthracycline

- Mismatch Repair:
  HNPCC → MSH_2
  MLH_1

  Endonucleases → Exonucleases → DNA polymerase → DNA Ligase → microsatellite
  Instability
- Base Excision Repair:
  Single base (depurination of DNA)
  N-Glycosylase (remove) → Nucleases → DNA Polymerases → DNA Ligases
- Nucleotide Excision-Repair:
  Less than 30 bp (<30 bp)
  Xeroderma pigmentosum (XP)
  Unwinding → Excision nucleases → DNA Polymerases → DNA Ligases
- Double-strand break repair:
  Proteins Ku and DNA-dependent protein kinase → combine to approximate the two strands and unwind → align → Base pair ligation

Histone—post translational modifications (RUPAM):

No poly 'A' tail for histone mRNA
R—**R**ibosylation (ADP)
U—**U**biquitination (SUMOylation—Small Ubiquitin-like Modifier)
P—**P**hosphorylation
A—**A**cetylation
M—**M**ethylation
NO glycosylation/NO oxidation/NO deamination

TRANSCRIPTION

ORI: Origin of Replication
Helicase: Unwinding (DNA)
DNA polymerase III: 5′ → 3′
DNA polymerase I: 5′ → 3′ Exonuclease
DNA ligase
SSB a nuclear protein (transcription termination factor) – protect DNA from nuclease

Lac operon (lactose operon):
Lac Z - β-galactosidase
Lac Y - Lactose permease
Lac A - Galactoside O-acetyltransferase (acetylase)
Lac I - Negative regulator (glucose +)
CRP - Positive regulator (No glucose)

[catabolite activator protein (CAP) and cyclic adenosine monophosphate (cAMP)]

Lactose – Inducer

IPTG – Gratuitous inhibitor

(Isopropyl-β-D-thiogalactoside)

TRANSCRIPTION Regulation protein

- **Helix turn**:
  - Lac repressor
  - Helix homeobox
  - MODY – 4
- **Zinc finger**: Steroid receptor
  - Thyroid
  - Waardenburg syndrome
  - WAGR syndrome - Wilms tumour (a tumour of the kidneys)
    - Aniridia (absence of the iris)
    - Genitourinary anomalies
    - Retardation.
- **Lucine Zipper**:
  - CREB (cAMP response element-binding protein)
  - Myc protein
  - Retinitis pigmentosa [AD] - neural retina leucine zipper (NRL)

hnRNA—Post-translational Modification

- Spleening of Exon
- Poly A – tail
- 5′ capping with methyl GTP
- Methylation
- (NO Phosphorylation/NO glycosylation)

Protein Targeting and Trafficking Defects

- Refsum disease
- Zellweger syndrome/Adrenoleukodystrophy (ALD)
- Primary hyperoxaluria
- Inclusion cell (I-cell) disease

Regan Isoenzyme

- Carcinoplacental isoenzyme of ALP
- Carcinoma of Lung/bone
- Smoking
- NADPH (Nicotinamide adenine dinucleotide phosphate):
  - MEOS Microsomal ethanol oxidizing system (chronic alcoholism)
  - Malic enzyme
  - Isocitrate dehydrogenase → *source*
  - HMP pathway
  - Aldose reductase (carbonyls)
  - Uronic acid pathway
  - Glutathione reductase
  - Fatty acid synthesis (no β oxidation)
  - Plasmalogen and PAF (Platelet-activating factor) synthesis

- Ceramide synthesis
- Cholesterol synthesis (not ketone synthesis)
- Bile acid synthesis
- Methemoglobin → hemoglobin
- Phenylalanine → Tyrosine

Fatty acid synthesis (enzymes cascade)

Ketoacyl synthase
↓
Ketoacyl reductase
↓
Hydroxyacyl dehydratase
↓ (H_2O)
Enoyl reductase
↓
Thioesterase/deacylase

β-Oxidation (enzymes cascade)

Acyl CoA synthase
↓
Acyl CoA dehydrogenase
↓
Hydratase
↓ (H_2O)
Dehydrogenase
↓
Thiolase

Ketone synthesis (substrate and enzymes cascade)

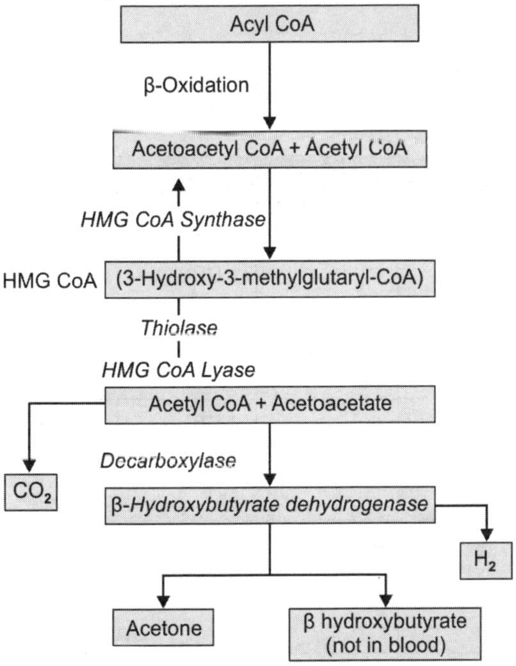

Trans → synthetic

Cis → MC in human body

Citrate lyase and HMG CoA reductase active in Phosphorylated form

Sphingolipids → NO Phosphorylation

Multiple Sclerosis → absent ethanol amine Plasmalogen and Sphingolipids from (From white matter of CNS)

$$\begin{array}{ccccc} 5 & 4 & 3 & 2 & 1 \\ \delta & \gamma & \beta & \downarrow\alpha & \\ CH_3- & CH_2- & CH_2- & CH_2- & COOH \\ \omega_1 & \omega_2 & \omega_3 & \omega_4 & \end{array}$$

β-Oxidation

Saturated

- BBC: Butter-Butyric acid (4C)
  Caproic acid (6C)
- CML: Coconut-Lauric acid (12C)
  Myristic acid (14C)
- BSP: Body-Stearic acid (18C)
  Palmitic acid (16C) —129 ATP

Unsaturated: (no human beyond Δ^9)

No. of Carbon	Fatty acid	ω nos.	Double bonds (DB)	Present in
18	Oleic acid	ω_9	1 DB	
18	Linoleic acid (most essential)	ω_6	2 DB	Safflower
18	Linolenic acid	ω_3- α ω_6 - β	3 DB	Soybean
20	Arachidonic acid	ω_6	4 DB	Meat, egg, milk
20	Timnodonic acid	ω_3	5 DB	Eicosapentaenoic acid (EPA) – fish oil
22	Cervonic acid	ω_3	6 DB	Docosahexaenoic acid (DHA) – breast milk In RP (retinitis pigmentosa)

Phospholipase Cleavage Sites

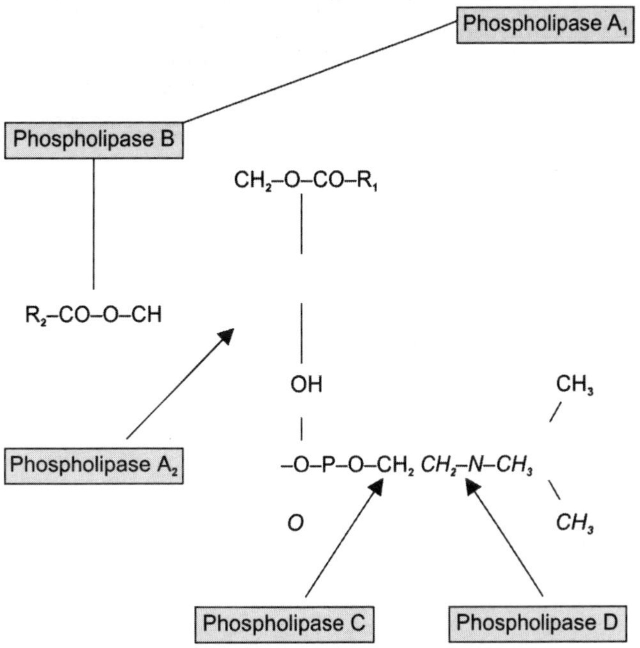

Phospholipase B = Phospholipase A_1 + Phospholipase A_2

Phospholipases

Phospholipase A_1		Acylglycerol, Phosphorylcholine + fatty acid
Phospholipase A_2	Snake venom, Pancrease	Lysolecithin + fatty acid
Phospholipase C	Bacterial tocin	1, 2 diacyl glycerol + Phosphorylcholine
Phospholipase D	Mammalian signal transducer	phosphatidic acid + choline

Sphingomyelin → sphingosine + choline; no sugar moiety

Sialic acid → N-acetylneuraminic acid (NANA) – gangliosides

Lecithin → phosphatidylcholine (PC)

Cephalin → Phosphatidylethanolamines (PEA)

Cardiolipin → Diphosphatidyl glycerol (DPG)

Ceramide → sphingosine + fatty acid; is present in cerebroside, gangliosides, Sphingomyelin

Surfactant

- Dipalmitoylphosphatidylcholine + DPPC
- Phosphatidylglycerol
- Cholesterol
- Surfactant A, B, C

VLDL → Endogenous lipoprotein and Triglycerides transport from liver
LDL → Has maximum cholesterol and cholesterol transport to peripheral tissue
HDL → α lipoprotein – no apo B

BILE ACID: (7alpha-dehydratase)	
1°	2°
Cholic acid Chenodeoxycholic acid and its taurine/glycine conjugate	Deoxycholic acid lithocholic acid and its taurine/glycine conjugate

Not Cross Cell Membrane

- Oxaloacetate
- Glucose 6 phosphate
- Acetyl CoA

apo B100 is one of the largest monomeric proteins of body

Titin is the largest known protein.

Prime – Pentose sugar L → R

Bond 3′→ 5′ (β-N glycosidic linkage)

Nucleotide 5′→ 3′ (5′ → PO_4) Sugar – use prime (prime sugar)

Transcription 5′→ 3′

'N' glycosidic

'O' glycosidic

Glycosidic → hemiacetal + alcohol/phenol

(non reducing)

Salvage → HGPRTase (recycling) – RBC and Brain Only salvage

Denovo – phosphoribosyl amidotransferase

Both – PRPP synthetase (preliminary step)

Soret band – 405 nm – Porphyrins

260 nm – Nucleotides

360 nm – Woods lamp

290 nm – Aromatic AA

Proline and Hydroxyproline, Chymoproline → no α helix

Collagen (collagen right handed helix) – Glycine > Proline

Dansyl Chloride – Determine number of polypeptide (PP) chains

Sanger's reagent – End group analysis

(1-fluoro-2, 4-dinitrobenzene)

Edman reagent – Protein sequencing

(phenylisothiocyanate (PITC))

Ingrams – Fingerprinting

Protein Structure

1° – Peptide bond (covalent)
2° – Hydrogen bond
3° – Hydrophobic interaction
4° – Disulphide and Hydrophobic
Super secondary → loops-helix-motiff
salting out – at high concentration solubility decreases
salting in – at low concentration solubility increases

Quantitative Protein Estimation

- Kjeldahl method
- Biuret method
- Lowry method
- Spectrophotometer
- Mancini (radial immunodiffusion)
- Nephelometry
- Turbidimetry (Sulfosalicylic acid)

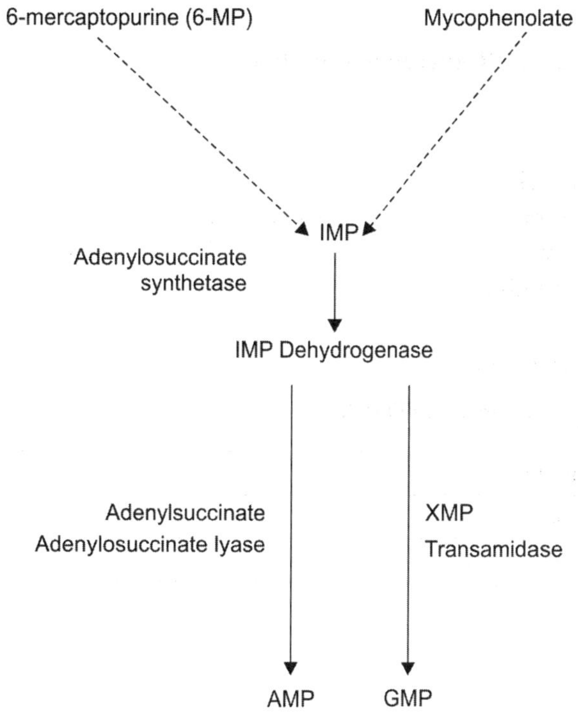

Catabolism: AIHXU
- Adenosine (A)
- Inosine (I)
- Hypoxanthine (H)
- Xanthine (X)
- Uric acid (U).

5-fluorouracil (5FU) × Thymidylate synthase

Allopurinol × Xanthine oxidase (molybdenum)
(suicide inhibitor)

5-Phosphoribosyl 1-pyrophosphate (PRPP)
Azaserine (1 and 4) × PRPP amido transferase (Glutamine → Glutamate + PPi)
5 phosphoribosylamine

Heme —(Heme oxygenase)→ Biliverdin —(Biliverdin reductase)→ Bilirubin

Deoxy – Taut (T) – Low affinity
Oxy – Relaxed (R) – High affinity

PING-PONG mechanism: Product released prior attach of another substrate
(Bi-Bi)

Amino transferase
Serine protease
→ Double – Replacement reaction

Serine protease →
Trypsin
Chymotrypsin (no pepsin)
Elastase
Thrombin

Allopurinol – vitamin B_{12} (orotic aciduria)

Folinic acid → N^5-formyl-tetrahydrofolic acid (THFA)

Glycine + Succinyl CoA = Porphyrin synthesis
Arginine + Glycine = Creatine synthesis
Homocysteine + Serine = Cystathionine = Homoserine + Cysteine

Gel filtration chromatography:

- Molecular size (stokes radius)
- Exclusion chromatography

Affinity chromatography:

- High selectivity
- Enzymes
- Urea
- Guanidine

Mass spectrometry:

- 1° structure
- Post translational modification

Chromosome walking:

- Sequencing

Microarray:

- Gene expression

Ion Exchange Chromatography

- Cation-exchange-chromatography: Positively charged molecules moves slow (carboxy alleles)
- Anion-exchange-chromatography: Negatively charged molecules moves slow (diethylaminoethanol {DEAE})

SDS (anionic) – PAGE

Sodium dodecyl sulfate (SDS) - PolyAcrylamide Gel Electrophoresis (PAGE)
- Molecular weight
- 1 SDS for 2 Peptide bond
- Purity of Protein

FAD-involving enzymes: (flavin adenine dinucleotide):
- Dihydrolipoyl dehydrogenase (in Pyruvate dehydrogenase complex PDH)
- Succinate dehydrogenase
- α - ketoglutarate dehydrogenase
- Glycerol 3 phosphate dehydrogenase shuttle
- Thioredoxin reductase (nucleotide)
- Glycolate oxidase
- Acyl CoA dehydrogenase (β Oxidation)

Meister's cycle or *Gamma-glutamyl cycle:*
Absorption of ATP in brain, intestine, kidney
Uses 3 ATP

Garrod's tetrad: Tetrad comprises four inherited metabolic diseases

Folic acid deficiency: Formiminoglutamic acid (FIGLU) excretion in urine

Miminoglutamic acid

Nonessential amino acid: (No GAPST)

3 PO_4 glycerate → Serine ← → Glycine

Choline ← (from Glycine)

α ketoglutarate	Glutamate	→
Pyruvate	Alanine	→
Oxaloacetate	Aspartate	→
L-Glutamate	Proline	→
Phenylalanine	Tyrosine	→

Tryptophan	**Glycine**
Niacin	Creatinine
Melatonin	Haeme
Seratonin	

Aromatic amino acid – UV light 290 nm

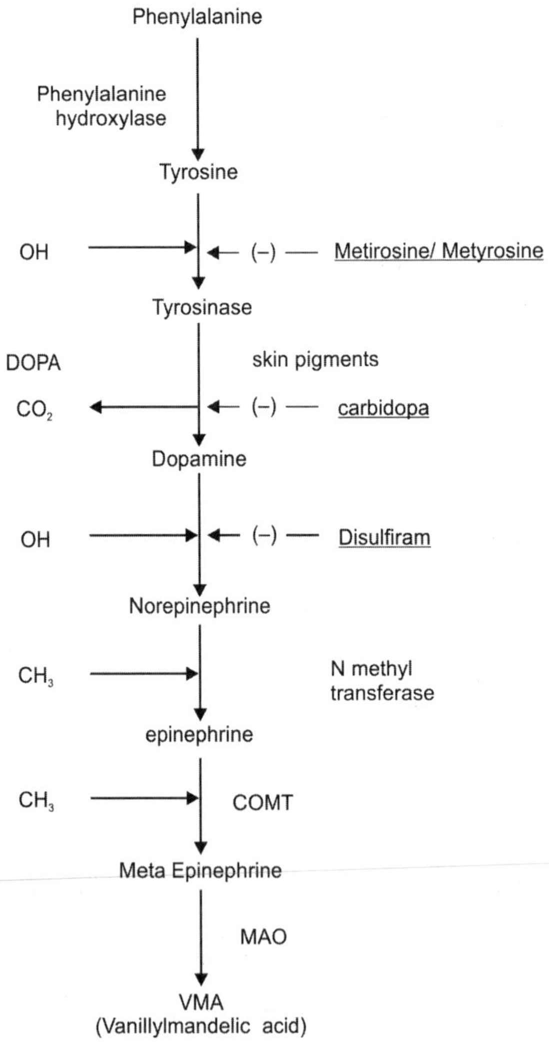

gamma-Glutamyl, cysteinyl, glycine → Glutathione

Melanin ----------- Tyrosine
Melatonin -------- Tryptophan

Suicide Inhibitors

- Allopurinol
- Aspirin cyclooxygenase
- Ornithine decarboxylase
- 5 FU

	Aldehyde	Ketone
Tetroses	Erythrose	Erythrulose
Pentoses	Arabinose Ribose Xylose	Ribulose Xylulose

Anomer: $\alpha_1 \beta$ 1st carbon

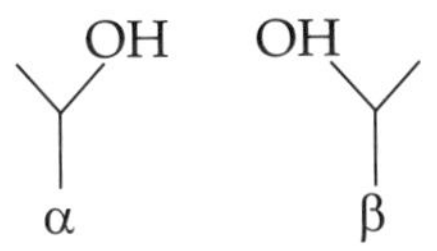

Epimer:
1st and Penultimate in glucose
2nd Mannose and 4th Galactose

Enantiomer: D, L mirror image with Penultimate carbon

Optical activity: d (+), l (–)

Hemiacetal - Fischer formula
Pyranose - Howarth formula

Zinc:
- Xanthine oxidase
- Carbonic anhydrase

Magnesium:
- Kinase
- Peptidase

Copper:
- Tyrosinase
- Superoxide dismutase
- Amine oxidase
- Cytochrome oxidase

Calcium:
- Lecithinase
- Lipase

Alcohol dehydrogenase:
- Carboxypeptidase
- Superoxide dismutase
- ALP
- RNA polymerase

BIOCHEMICAL TESTS

Carbohydrates

- Reducing sugar – *Benedict's test/Fehling's test*
- Monosaccharides – *Barfoed's test*
- Fructose – *Seliwanoff's test/Foulger's test*
- 5-Carbon (Pentoses) – Molisch test – furfural

Protein

- Nitric acid – *heller's test*
- Amino acid – Acid heat *NINHYDRIN* test
- 2 Peptide bonds – *Biuret test*
- Phenol gp – *Millon's test* (specific for tyrosine, not Phenylalanine)
- Phenylalanine, Tyrosine, Tryptophan: Benzene ring—*Xanthoproteic test*
- Tryptophan (indole) – *Aldehyde test (Hopkins-Cole)*
- Arginine (guanidine) – *Sakaguchi's test*
- SH-gp – *Nitroprusside test* (specific for cysteine–homocystinuria)
- Imidazole and tyrosine – *Pauly test*

Bile Pigment

- Fouchet's test
- Gmelin's test
- Van den Bergh test
- Ehrlich's test (urobilinogen)

Bile Salt

- Pettenkofer's test
- Hay's test

Ketone

- Acetoacetic acid – *Gerhardt's test* ($FeCl_3$)
- Acetone + Acetoacetic acid – *Rothera's Nitroprusside* test

Urobilinogen

- Ehrlich's test
- Schlesinger's test
- Phenylketonuria: Guthrie test (neonatal heel prick test)
- Phenylketonuria and Alkaptonuria: $FeCl_3$ test (ferric chloride)
- Galactosuria: Mucic Acid
- Folic Acid Deficiency: Figlu (Formiminoglutamic acid)
- Hartnup's Disease: Obermeyer test
- Tyrosinemia: Nitrosonaphthol test
- Essential Pentosuria: Bial's test
- DNA: Feulgen stain
- MSUD (Maple syrup urine disease): DNPH (**2, 4**-dinitrophenylhydrazine)

CONCEPTS IN BIOCHEMISTRY

- Rate-limiting step:

First irreversible step
Unique to that cycle

- Those enzymes which act in well fed state (anabolic) will be in dephosphorylated form and those in fasting(catabolic) state – will be in phosphoylated form, e.g. glycogen synthase active in dephosphorylated form.
- Enzymes containing 'tase' involves ATP, e.g. phosphatase
- Fat cannot be converted to carbohydrate, i.e. Acetyl CoA cannot be converted to Glucose as pyruvate to acetyl CoA step is irrevesibe. But carbohydrates can be converted to fat.
- But 'Fats are burned at fire of carbohydrate', i.e. fatty acid oxidation need ATP.
- Glucose-6-phosphatase is present only in liver so only liver can do gluconeogenesis.
- Glutamate dehydrogenase is available only in liver so urea cycle occurs in liver
- Glycerol kinase absent in muscle and adipose tissue so no esterification in adipose tissue
- Mitochondria is impermeable to oxaloacetate and acetyl CoA—hence the malate shuttle exists.

Ping-pong reaction:

First substrate is bound and its product release prior to the binding of the second substrate, e.g. aminotransferases and serine proteases.

Bi-Bi reactions:

Two substrate and two product reactions

***Amphibolic pathways*:**

Reactions that link between the catabolic and anabolic pathways, e.g. Citric acid cycle.

Anaplerotic reactions:

Otherwise called as filling up reactions. Substrates moves in and out, e.g Pyruvate carboxylase

Cotranslational insertion:

The insertion of the signal peptide into the conducting channel, while the other end of the parent protein is still attached to ribosomes.

Mass spectroscopy detects primary structure and posttranslational modifications of proteins

Only L-Amino acids are present in human proteins

Strong acid – low pKA

Stone	Shape	Radio-opacity	Formed in
Calcium oxalate Calcium PO4	Octahedron	Opaque	Acidic urine
Struvite	Coffin lid	Opaque	Alkaline urine
Uric acid	Rhomboid	Radiolucent	
Cysteine	Hexagonal	Opaque	Acidic urine

GENETICS

Glossary

- Genetic heterogeneity: Mutations in several genetic loci producing same trait, e.g. profound childhood deafness.
- Pleotrophism: Single gene defect causing multiple unrelated problems, e.g. Sickle cell.
- Variable expressivity: Same defect with different phenotypic spectrum in affected individuals, e.g. Alzeimer's disease and MEN
- Degeneracy/Redundancy: Same amino acid coded by many codons.
- Chimerism: Showing cell lines from two different zygotes
- Mosaicism: Genetically different cell types arising from a single zygote.
- Gonadal mosaicism: In autosomal dominant disorders mutation occurring only in gonads, so their children are not affected.
- Codominance: Fully expressed in heterogeneous state, e.g. ABO blood group antigens
- Genetic mutation: Change in chromosome numbers, loss or gain of whole chromosome.
- Chromosomal mutation: Rearrangement within the chromosome giving rise to visible structural changes.
- Genomic imprinting: Selective deletion, e.g. deletion of paternal chr 22 – Prader Willi syndrome, deletion of maternal chr 22 – Angelman syndrome.
- Uniparental disomy: Both alleles derived from a same parent – Autosomal recessive.
- Epigenetics: Chemical modification of the genes which does not alter DNA sequencing, e.g. Methylation and acetylation.

CHAPTER 6 Microbiology

Spot Check

Shangai fever	Pseudomonas
Whirlpool fever	Pseudomonas
Jacuzzi fever	Pseudomonas
Pontiac fever	Legionella
Malta fever	Brucella
Undulant fever	Brucella
Glander	B. malli
Melioidosis	B. pseudomallei (great imitator of syphilis)
3-day fever	Sandfly fever
5-day fever	B. quintana (trench fever)
Ratbite fever	Spirillum minus, streptobacillus moniliformis
8-day disease	Tetanus neonatorum
Fitz-High-Curtis syndrome	Gonococci, Chlamydia
Brazilian purpuric fever	H.aegypticus
Circling disease	Listeria meningitidis
Oroya fever	Bartonella
Carrion's disease	Bartonella basilliformis
Cat-scratch disease	Bartonella henselae
Red-Leg disease	Aeromonas
Chigger typhus	Scrub
Yaws	T. pertunae
Pinta	T. carateum
Eaton agent	Mycoplasma
Whitmore bacillus	B. pseudomallei
Friedlander bacillus	Klebsiella
Pfeiffer	H. influenza
Kochweek	H. aegypticus
Axenfeld	Moraxella lacunata
Kanagawa phenomenon	V. parahemolyticus
Medusa	B. anthrax
Nagler's	Cl. perfringens
Chinese letter pattern	Cuneiform bacillus

Drumstick terminal	Cl. tetani
Subterminal bulging	Cl. botulinum
Anton test	Losteria
String test	Vibrio cholerae
Castaneda method	Brucella, salmonella
PPAR	Proteus
Citron body	C. psittaci

Dimorphic Fungi

- Candida albicans
- Histoplasma capsulatum
- Sporothrix
- Blastomycosis
- Coccidomycosis, paracoccidomycosis
- Penicillium

Acid Fast

- Mycobacterium
- Nocardia
- Cyclospora
- Rhodococcus
- Spermatic head
- Legionella
- Lepra bacillus
- Isospora
- Cryptosporidium
- Smegma bacillus
- Bacterial spores
- Egg of T. saginata

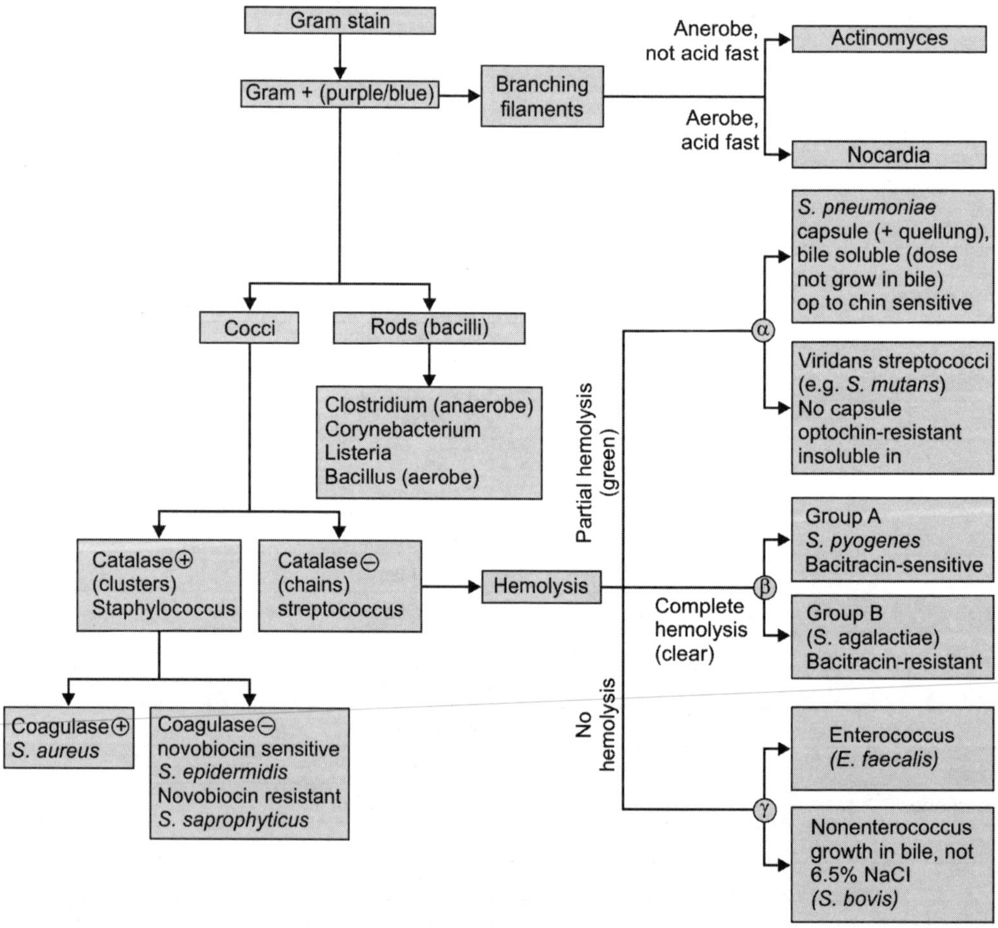

TOXIN

- Cholera toxin-activate adenyl cyclase-increase cAMP (Gs, alpha subunit)
- ETEC heat stable toxin-activate guanyl cyclase-increase cGMP
- Pertussis toxin-inhibit adenyl cyclase-increase cAMP

Microaerophilic

- Campylobacter
- Borrelia burgdorferri
- Spirochetes
- H. pylori
- Streptococcus

BIOFILM

- CONS
- Strep. mutans (dental extraction)
- Staph. aureus

Autoinfection *(CCHETS)*

- Cryptosporidium
- Hymenolepsis nana
- Taenia solium
- Capillaria philippinensis
- Enterobius
- Strongyloides

Obligate anerobes	Clostridium, bacteroides
Microaerophilic	Streptococci, spirochaetes

Motile

- All enterobacteria ***except Klebsiella, Shigella***
- Proteus
- Vibrio
- Campylobacter
- Clostridium ***except C. perfringens and tetani***
- Burkholderia pseudomallei
- Campylobacter
- Pseudomonas
- Salmonella ***except S. gallinarum***
- Bacillus
- Legionella
- Yersinia enterocolitica
- Listeria at ***25 degrees centigrade***

Capsulated

- B. anthrax
- Cl. perfringens
- Pneumococcus
- H. influenzae
- V. cholerae 0139
- V. parahemolyticus
- Bordetella
- Neisseria
- Klebsiella

Safety Pin

- Brucella
- Burkholderia pseudomallei
- V. parahemolyticus
- Calymmatobacterium
- Bordetella
- Yersinia
- H. ducreyi

Intracellular

- Brucella
- Legionella
- Chlamydia
- M. leprae
- N. gonorrhea
- Listeria
- Ricketssia except R. quintana
- Yersinia

Blood-borne Infections

- Hepatitis B, C, G
- HTLV 1
- Parvovirus B 19
- HIV 1
- CMV

Strict Aerobe

- Vibrio
- Pseudomonas
- M. tuberculosis

Swarming

- Cl. tetani
- B. cereus
- P. vulgaris
- P. mirabilis

Anaerobes

Gram-positive cocci	Peptostreptococcus, peptococcus
Gram-negative cocci	Veillonella
Gram-positive bacilli	Eubacterium, Propionibacterium, Actinomyces, Lactobacilli, Mobiluncus, Bifidobacterium
Gram-negative bacillus	Bacteroides, prevotella, pyromonas, fusobacterium, leptotrium

Lactose fermenters	E. coli, Klebsiella, Staph enterococci, citrobacter
Late lactose fermenters	Shigella sonnei, Vibrio cholerae
Nonlactose fermenters	Salmonella, shigella, EIEC, proteus

Shigella dysenteriae	No mannitol fermenting, exotoxin

Components Involved in Molecular Mimicry

Capsular hyaluronic acid	Synovial fluid
Cell wall protein	Myocardium
Group A carbohydrate	Cardiac valves
Cytoplasmic membrane antigen	Vascular
Peptidoglycans	Skin antigen

Urease test positive: H. pylori > proteus > klebsiella > citro
Oxidase positive: Neisseria, Pseudomonas, Vibro, Haemophilus, Aeromonas, Bordetella, Brucella, Campylobacter
Catalase positive: Staphylococci, Pseudomonas, Vibrio, Haemophilus, Shigella, Bordetella, E. coli, Campylobacter

Streptococcus:

Group	Organism
A	S. pyogenes
B	S. agalactiae
C	S. equisimilus (ribose-fermenting) (capsulated)
D	Enterococci
Nontyped	Viridans

EPEC Enteroadherent E. coli

- Diarrhea in infants
- BFP: Bundle-forming pilli

ETEC

- Traveller's diarrhea
- Heat-labile: cAMP
- Heat-stable: cGMP

EIEC

- Nonlactose fermentor
- Sereney test
- VMA (virulence marker antigen)
- Nonmotile

EHEC = STEC = VTEC

- HUS sorbitol fermenting
- 0157: H7
- RIP: Ribosome inhibiting protein
- Phage-mediated

Nontoxin-mediated: EPEC, EOEC

EAEC

- Chronic diarrhea, persistent diarrhea, traveler's diarrhea.

S. dysenteriae	Group A
S. flexneri	B
S. boydii	C (India)
S. sonnei	D

Plague vectors

North India	X. cheopsis
South India	X. astia

Salmonella

Somatic O	> 1/100, heat-stable, granular, round
Flagella H	> 1/200, most immunogenic, fluffy, conical tube VI carrier

Colony appearances

- Raindrop colony: Bordetella
- Honeydrop colony: Brucella

- Oil paint appearance: Staph
- Aluminum paint: Bordetella

El-tor Vibrio

- Polymyxin, phage IV resistance
- VP, hemolysin, chick RBC agglutination

Eschar

- Rickettsialpox
- Scrub typhus

Endotoxin produced by **Gram positive**	Listeria
Exotoxin produced by **Gram negative**	Shiga toxin
Typhus Fevers:	
Epidemic typhus	R. prowazekii, Brill-Zinsser disease, Red louse disease
Endemic typhus	R. typhi, Neil Mooser Rn

Neil Mooser +	Endemic typhus
Hide porter	Cutaneous anthrax
Wool sorter	Pulmonary anthrax
OX – Z–	Rocky mountain spotted fever
OX – K–	Scrub typhus (OX-19) negative

TB

Niacin, nitrate reduction	Human
Neutral red	Virulent
Aryl sulfatase, catalase	Atypical
Catalase mutation	INH-resistant

Sterilization Control

B. stearothermophilus	Autoclaving
B. globigii	ETO sterilization
B. subtilis	Ionizing radiation
C. tetani	Hot air oven

HPV

1	Plantar wart
6, 11	Condyloma accuminata/Laryngeal papilloma
16, 18, 33, 45	CA cervix
18	Adeno CA cervix
2, 7	Palmar/Butcher wart

Dead-end host infections

- Leptospira
- Tetanus
- Human rabies
- Echinococcus
- Brucella
- Legionella
- Endemic typhus
- T. solium
- Trichinella spiralis
- Bubonic plague

Bacteria	Medium
Staph	Ludlam's, salt-milk, RCM, nutrient agar
Streptococcus	Sheep blood agar, pikes transport
Corynebacterium	Loeffler's slope, tellurite blood agar
Bacillus anthracis	PLET
B. cereus	MYPA
Legionella	BCYE
Listeria	Thioglycolate broth
Gonococcus	Thayer-Martin medium
Meningococcus	Modified Thayer-Martin medium
E. coli	MacConkey agar
Salmonella	Selenite F broth
Shigella	Deoxycholate citrate agar
Francisella	Francis blood dextrose cysteine agar
Vibrio	TCBS, Mansour's GTA, alkaline bile salt, alkaline peptone water
V. parahaemolyticus	Nagatsuma agar
Pseudomonas	Cetrimide agar
Haemophilus	Chocolate agar
Bordetella	Bordet-Gengou potato glycerine blood agar
Campylobacter	Skirrow's, Butzler's, Campy-BAP
Borrelia	BSK: Barbour-Stoenner-Kelly
Brucella	Castaneda method
Yersinia	CIN medium
Leptospira	EMJH, Fletcher, Korthoff, Stuart
TB	Solid: LJ and dorset Liquid: Dubo and Middlebrook
Fastidious cocci	Brain-heart infusion broth
Trichomonas	CPLM medium
Leishmania and trypanosoma	NNN
Anerobes	RCM
Acanthamoeba	Nutrient agar with E. coli

Continuous Cell Lines

- *Hela*: Human CA cervix cell line
- *Hepa*: Human epithelioma larynx
- *KB*: Human CA nasopharynx
- *MCCOY*: Human synovial carcinoma
- *Vero*: Vervet monkey kidney

PHAGE TYPING

- Salmonella
- Staph. aureus
- Diphtheria
- V. cholera
- B. anthrax

Premunition

- Syphilis
- Malaria

Enterovirus

70	Acute hemorrhagic conjunctivitis
71	Hand-Foot-Mouth
72	Hepatitis A

COMMON COLD

- Rhino
- Adeno
- Corona (SARS)
- Parainfluenza

DNA Virus

- Papova-papilloma, polyoma
- Pox
- Hepadna
- *All RNA viruses SS except Reoviridae*
- Parvo
- Herpes
- Adeno
- *All DNA viruses DS except Parvovirus*

SMALLEST AND LARGEST

Smallest RNA Picorna
Smallest DNA Parvo
Largest RNA Paramyxo
Largest DNA Pox

Enveloped DNA virus

All except:

- Parvo
- Papova
- Adeno

Enveloped RNA virus

All except:

- Picorna
- Calici
- Rheo

Positive sense:

- Picarno
- Calici
- Flavi
- Corona
- Toga

Negative sense

RNA Virus

- **Segmented**
  - Buniya (hanta)
  - Orthomyxo
  - Reo (rota)
  - Arena (lassa)
- **Nonsegmented**
  - Rhabdo
  - Paramyxo
  - Filoviridae

LIVE VACCINES

Measles	Edmonston-Zagreb
Mumps	Jeryl Lynn
Rubella	RA 27/3
Varicella	Oka
Yellow fever	17 D, Asibi
BCG	Danish 133
Polio	Sabin
JE	SA 14, 14, 2

Diarrhea and Viruses

- Group A Rota virus
- Noro virus (Norwalk)
- Sapovirus (Caliciviridae)
- Astrovirus
- Corona virus

Hepatitis

A	Picarno
B	Hepadna
C and G	Flaviviridae
D	Delta virus (defective)
E	Calicivirus

Arbovirus

Togaviridae	Alphavirus (Group A), Chikungunya, sindbis
Flaviviridae	Group B
Mosquito	Dengue, JE, yellow fever
Tick	KFD, West Nile fever
Bunyaviridae	Buniyavirus
Phlebo	Sandfly, Rift Valley fever
Nairo	Ganjan
Hanta	Hanta, puumala
Rheoviridae	Orbivirus, African horse sickness, colorado tick
Rhabdoviridae	Vesicular stomatitis, Rabies
Filoviridae	Ebola, Marburg

Inclusion Bodies

Cytoplasm:

Negri	Rabies
Vaccinia	Guarneri
Fowlpox	Bollinger
Molluscum	Henderson-Peterson
Smallpox	Paschen
Chlamydia	HP

Heterophiles:

Mycoplasma: O blood group
EBV: Sheep RBCs
Protein: Rickettsia

Mycobacterium tuberculosis complex:

M. tuberculosis
M. bovis
M. africanum
M. microti

EBV-associated Ca:

- Tonsil Ca
- Angioimmunoblastic lymphadenopathy
- Angiocentric NK/T cell
- T cell lymphoma
- Thymoma
- CNS lymphoma
- Gastric Ca

Nucleus:

- Cowdry A: Herpes Lipshutz, Yellow: Torre
- Cowdry B: Adeno (basophilic), Polio
- Miyagawa bodies: Chlamydia trachomatis infection
- Lafora bodies: Familial myoclonic epilepsy
- Tuffstone bodies: Metachromatic leukodystrophy

Yaws:

- Frambosie
- Crab yaw
- Relapse common

Endemic syphilis:

- Mouth-mouth
- Mucocutaneous

Pinta:

- Pruritic
- Papule
- Dyschromic macule

Caseous necrosis:

- TB
- Syphilis
- Histoplasmosis
- Coccidiomycosis

Tuberculids:

- Lichen scrofulosorum
- Erythema induratum
- Acne scrofulaceum
- Rosacea tuberculids

ATYPICAL TUBERCULOUS ORGANISMS

Photochromogen	M. kansasii, marinum
Scotochromogen	M. scrofulaceum
Nonphotochromogen	M. intracellulare, avium, ulcerans
Rapid growers	M. fortium, smegmatis, vaccae

HIV

Gag	p24
Pol	p31
Env	gp 160 (41+120)

Vectors

Epidemic typhus	R. prowazeki	Louse
Endemic typhus	R. typhi	Rat flea
Scrub typhus	R. tsutsugamushi	Trombiculid mite
Indian tick typhus	R. conorii	Tick
Rocky mountain spotted fever	R. rickettsii	Tick
Rickettsialpox	R. akari	Gamasid mite
Q fever	C. burnetii	Soft tick
Trench fever	Rochalimaea quintana	Louse

FUNGAL SPORES

Basidiopore: Cryptococcus
Chlamydospore: Candida
Arthroconidia: Coccidiomycosis
Blastoconidia: Blastomycosis

Hypesensitivity Reactions

Type 1

- Casoni
- Prausnitz-Küstner
- Asthma
- Anaphylaxis
- Shultz-Dale
- Theobald Smith
- Eczema
- Urticaria

Type 2

- Blood transfusion
- Erythroblastosis fetalis
- Pernicious anemia
- Graves
- AIHA, ITP
- Goodpasture
- ARF
- Myasthenia

Type 3

- Schick test
- PSGN
- SLE
- HSP
- Farmer's lung, ABPA (also 1)
- Arthus/serum sickness
- PAN
- ENL
- Hypersensitive pneumonitis (also 4)

Type 4

- Frie's test
- Lepromin/tuberculin
- Contact dermatitis
- Temporal arteritis
- GBS
- Fairley's test (schistosomiasis)
- Patch test
- Graft rejection
- Multiple sclerosis

Concepts and Facts

- The most virulent of the genus, Staphylococcus aureus, is one of the most common causes of bacterial infections, and is also an important cause of food poisoning and toxic shock syndrome.
- Staphylococcus epidermidis is an important cause of prosthetic implant infections, whereas Staphylococcus saprophyticus causes urinary tract infections, especially cystitis in women.
- Generally, significant host compromise is required for S. aureus infection, such as a break in the skin or insertion of a foreign body (for example, wounds, surgical infections, or central venous catheters), an obstructed hair follicle (folliculitis), or a compromised immune system.
- Enterotoxins (six major antigenic types: A, B, C, D, E, and G) are produced by approximately half of all S. aureus isolates.
- Toxic shock syndrome toxin is the classic cause of toxic shock syndrome. Because of similarities in molecular structure, it is sometimes referred to as staphylococcal enterotoxin F (SEF), although it does not cause food poisoning when ingested.
- The most common S. aureus infections are small, superficial abscesses involving hair follicles (folliculitis) or sweat or sebaceous glands. For example, the common sty (external hordeolum) is created by infection of an eyelash follicle.
- Subcutaneous abscesses called furuncles (boils) often form around foreign bodies, such as splinters. These generally respond to local therapy, that is, removal of the foreign body, soaking, and drainage as indicated.
- Carbuncles are larger, deeper, multiloculated skin infections that can lead to bacteremia and require antibiotic therapy and debridement.

- Impetigo is usually a localized, superficial, spreading crusty skin lesion generally seen in children. It can be caused by S. aureus, although more commonly by Streptococcus pyogenes, or both organisms together.
- The incidence of vancomycin resistance has increased steadily, prompting the use of alternative drugs, such as quinupristin-dalfopristin, linezolid, and daptomycin. These agents have good in vitro activity against MRSA and most other clinically important gram-positive bacterial pathogens.
- S. saprophyticus can be distinguished from S. epidermidis and most other coagulase-negative staphylococci by its natural resistance to novobiocin.
- Streptococci are gram-positive, nonmotile, and catalase-negative.
- Diseases caused by this group of organisms include acute infections of throat and skin caused by Group A streptococci (Streptococcus pyogenes); female genital tract colonization, resulting in neonatal sepsis caused by Group B streptococci (Streptococcus agalactiae); pneumonia, otitis media, and meningitis caused by Streptococcus pneumoniae; and endocarditis caused by the viridans group of streptococci.
- The Lancefield scheme classifies primarily β-hemolytic streptococci into Groups A through U on the basis of their C-carbohydrate. The clinically most important groups of β-hemolytic streptococci are types A and B.
- Hyaluronic acid, identical to that found in human connective tissue, forms the outermost layer of the cell in a Group A streptococcus – Streptococcus pyogenes. This capsule is not recognized as foreign by the body and, therefore, is nonimmunogenic.
- Group A-specific C-carbohydrate is composed of rhamnose and N-acetylglucosamine.
  [Note: All Group A streptococci, by definition, contain this antigen].
- Protein F (fibronectin-binding protein) mediates attachment to fibronectin in the pharyngeal epithelium.
- S. pyogenes cells, perhaps in an inhaled droplet, attach to the pharyngeal mucosa via actions of protein F, lipoteichoic acid, and M protein.
- Impetigo is treated with a topical agent, such as mupirocin, or systemically with penicillin or a first-generation cephalosporin, such as cephalexin, which are effective against both S. aureus and S. pyogenes.
- Rapid latex antigen kits for direct detection of group A streptococci in patient samples are widely used. (They say latex test is for encapsulated bacteriae, group A is obviously one of them.)
- S. pyogenes has not acquired resistance to penicillin G, which remains the antibiotic of choice for acute streptococcal disease. In a penicillin-allergic patient, a macrolide such as clarithromycin or azithromycin is the preferred drug. Penicillin G plus clindamycin are used in treating necrotizing fasciitis and in streptococcal toxic shock syndrome.
- Group B streptococci, represented by the pathogen S. agalactiae, are gram-positive, catalase-negative organisms.
- Group B streptococci are a leading cause of meningitis and septicemia in neonates, with a high mortality rate.
- Group B streptococci are β-hemolytic, with larger colonies and less hemolysis than group A.
- Most isolates of streptococci (group B in β-hemolytic) remain sensitive to penicillin G and ampicillin, which are still the antibiotics of choice. In life-threatening infections, an aminoglycoside can be added to the regimen. [Note: Pregnant carriers should be treated with ampicillin during labor if risk factors such as premature rupture of membranes or prolonged labor are present.]
- S. pneumoniae are gram-positive, nonmotile, encapsulated cocci. They are lancet-shaped, and their tendency to occur in pairs accounts for their earlier designation as Diplococcus pneumoniae.
- S. pneumoniae is the most common cause of pneumonia and otitis media and an important cause of meningitis and bacteremia/sepsis.
- Patients with sickle cell disease or those who have had their spleens removed are particularly at risk for S. pneumoniae infection.
- The bacterial capsule of S. pneumoniae is the most important virulence factor, and is the basis for the classification of serotypes of this organism. Cell-associated enzymes, pneumolysin, and autolysin contribute to its pathogenicity.
- Mechanisms by which virus infection predisposes an individual to streptococcal pneumonia include increased volume and viscosity of secretions that are more difficult to clear and secondary inhibition of the action of bronchial cilia by viral infection.

- Otitis media is the most common bacterial infection of children (which is characterized by earache). It is most frequently caused by pneumococcus, followed by Haemophilus influenza and Moraxella catarrhalis.
- Bacteremia/sepsis in the absence of a focus of infection is commonly caused by pneumococcus, especially in splenectomized individuals.
- H. influenzae was formerly the leading cause of bacterial meningitis in the United States. After a vaccine was developed against this organism, S. pneumoniae became the most common cause of bacterial meningitis. This disease has a high mortality rate, even when treated appropriately.
- Most resistant strains of S. pneumoniae remain sensitive to third-generation cephalosporins (such as cefotaxime or ceftriaxone), and all are still sensitive to vancomycin; these antibiotics are therefore the agents of choice for invasive infections by penicillin-resistant strains of S. pneumoniae.
- Enterococci contain a C-carbohydrate that reacts with group D antisera.
- Enterococci are distinguished from the nonenterococcol Group D streptococci by their ability to survive in the presence of bile, and to hydrolyze the polysaccharide esculin. Unlike nonenterococcal group D streptococci, enterococci grow in 6.5 percent NaCl, and yield a positive pyrazin amidase (PYR) test. E. faecalis can be distinguished from E. faecium by their fermentation patterns, which are commonly evaluated in clinical laboratories.
- Streptococcus bovis is the most clinically important of the nonenterococcus group D streptococci.
- Corynebacteria are small, slender, pleomorphic, gram-positive rods of distinctive morphology that tend to stain unevenly.
- Diphtheria is caused by the local and systemic effects of a single exotoxin that inhibits eukaryotic protein synthesis by its action on Elongation Factor 2 (EF-2).
- Diphtheria consists of a strictly local infection, usually of the throat. The infection produces a distinctive thick, grayish, adherent exudate (pseudomembrane) that is composed of cell debris from the mucosa and inflammatory products.
- Although all human cells are sensitive to diphtheria toxin, the major clinical effects involve the heart and peripheral nerves.
- C. diphtheriae can be isolated most easily from a selective medium, such as Tinsdale's agar, which contains potassium tellurite, an inhibitor of other respiratory flora, and on which the organism produces several distinctive black colonies with halos. (TELL UR InTErn)
- Species of the genus Bacillus are gram-positive, form endospores, and are either strictly or facultatively aerobic (that is, they can grow in the presence of oxygen, but do not require it).
- B. anthracis possesses a capsule that is antiphagocytic and is essential for full virulence. The organism also produces three plasmid-coded exotoxins: edema factor, a calmodulin-dependent adenylate cyclase, causes elevation of intracellular cAMP, and is responsible for the severe edema usually seen in B. anthracis infections; lethal toxin is responsible for tissue necrosis; protective antigen (so named because of its use in producing protective anthrax vaccines) mediates cell entry of edema factor and lethal toxin.
- Microscopically, the organisms appear as blunt-ended bacilli that occur singly, in pairs, or frequently in long chains. They do not sporulate often in clinical samples, but do so in culture. The spores are oval and centrally located. On blood agar, the colonies are large, grayish, and nonhemolytic, with an irregular border. Unlike many bacillus species, B. anthracis is non-motile and is encapsulated in vivo. A direct immunofluorescence assay aids in identification of the organism.
- Listeria species are slender, short gram-positive rods. They do not form spores.
- Listeria species are catalase-positive (strep are catalase negative), and display a distinctive tumbling motility (corynebacterium are immotile) by light microscopy in liquid medium.
- L. monocytogenes is capable of growth at 4°C; thus refrigeration does not reliably suppress its growth in food.
- Septicemia and meningitis are the most commonly reported forms of L. monocytogenes infection (listeriosis).
- A variety of focal lesions are less frequently seen, such as granulomatous skin lesions. Pregnant women, usually in the third trimester, may have a milder flu-like illness. In this as well as in asymptomatic vaginal colonization, the organism can be transmitted to a newborn (L. monocytogenes is a relatively common cause of newborn meningitis) or to the fetus and initiate abortion.

- On blood agar, L. monocytogenes produces a small colony surrounded by a narrow zone of β hemolysis.
- Propionibacterium is a genus of anerobic or microaerophilic rods of diphtheroid-like morphology.
- P. acnes, often a strict anerobe, has been implicated as a contributing cause of acne.
- Erysipelothrix rhusiopathiae is a filamentous, gram-positive rod that causes disease in animals and, rarely, a skin infection called erysipeloid in people who commonly handle animal products, for example, butchers, veterinarians, and fishermen.
- The genus Neisseria consists of gram-negative, aerobic cocci.
- Gonococci are unencapsulated (unlike meningococci), piliated, and nonmotile, and resemble a pair of kidney beans.
- Gonococcal lipooligosaccharides (LOS) have shorter, more highly branched, nonrepeat O-antigenic side chains than do lipopolysaccharides found in other gram-negative bacteria.
- OMP II is referred to as the opacity protein because its presence renders gonococcal colonies less translucent. OMP II, along with pili, mediates attachment of the organism to a host cell.
- Most strains of gonococci have a limited ability to multiply in the bloodstream. Therefore, bacteremia with gonococci is rare. [Note: In contrast, meningococci multiply rapidly in blood]
- Gonococcal infection is the most common cause of septic arthritis in sexually active adults.
- N. gonorrhoeae grows best under aerobic conditions, and most strains require enhanced CO_2.
- N. gonorrhoeae ferments glucose but not maltose, lactose, or sucrose.
  [Note: N. meningitidis does ferment maltose]
- All members of the genus Neisseriae are oxidase-positive. A trick to remember the most medical-relevant oxidase positive bacteria is: 'Volatile Pressed Capsules Hide Nasty and Mean Looks' (*Vibrio, Pseudomonas, Campylobacter, Helicobacter, Neisseria, Moraxella,* and *Legionella,* respectively).
- Thayer-Martin medium (chocolate agar supplemented with several antibiotics that suppress the growth of nonpathogenic neisseriae and other normal and abnormal flora) is typically used to isolate gonococci.
- N. meningitidis tends to strike young, previously well individuals and can progress over a matter of hours to death.
- The LOS capsule is antigenically diverse, which allows the identification of at least fourteen capsular polysaccharide types, called serogroups.
- A second classification system called serotyping is also a serologic classification that is based on the properties of the outer membrane proteins and LOS.
- Petechial rash and neck extension are characteristic of meningococcal meningitis, or for that matter, any meningitis.
- Within several hours, the initial fever and malaise can evolve into severe headache, a rigid neck, vomiting, and sensitivity to bright lights, symptoms characteristic of meningitis. Coma can occur within a few hours.
- Acute, fulminating meningococcal septicemia seen mainly in very young children (the Waterhouse-Friderichsen syndrome). It is characterized by large, purple, blotchy skin hemorrhages, vomiting and diarrhea, circulatory collapse, necrosis of the adrenals, and death within ten to twelve hours.
- The gold standard for diagnosis of systemic meningococcal infection is the isolation of N. meningitidis from an usually sterile body fluid, such as blood or cerebrospinal fluid (CSF). In performing a Gram stain on CSF, the clinical sample is centrifuged to concentrate the organisms, because 10^5 to 10^6 bacteria per ml are required for this test.
- N. meningitidis ferments both glucose and maltose, whereas N. gonorrhoeae ferments only glucose.
- Members of the genus Moraxella are nonmotile, gram-negative coccobacilli that are generally found in pairs. Moraxella are aerobic, oxidase-positive, fastidious organisms that do not ferment carbohydrates. The most important pathogen in the genus is Moraxella (formerly, Branhamella) catarrhalis. This organism can cause infections of the respiratory system, middle ear, eye, CNS, and joints.
- Members of the genus Acinetobacter are nonmotile coccobacilli that are frequently confused with neisseriae in gram-stained samples. Generally encapsulated, oxidase-negative, and obligately aerobic, they do not ferment carbohydrates. They are important nosocomial (hospital-acquired) pathogens.

- Gram-negative bacterium do glucose fermentation test. Neisseriae are positive. Others are negative. Then do Oxidase test. Moraxella is positive. Acinetobacter is negative.
- Diseases caused by members of the genera Escherichia, Salmonella, Yersinia, and Campylobacter can be both gastrointestinal and extraintestinal, those caused by members of the genera Shigella, Helicobacter, and Vibrio are primarily gastrointestinal, and those caused by members of the genera Enterobacter, Klebsiella, Serratia, and Proteus are primarily extraintestinal.
- Most strains of E. coli can ferment lactose (that is, they are Lac^+) in contrast to the major intestinal pathogens, Salmonella and Shigella, which cannot ferment lactose (that is, they are Lac^-).
- E. coli shares many properties with the other Enterobacteriaceae. They are all true facultative anerobes. They all ferment glucose, and can generate energy by reducing nitrates to nitrites. They all lack cytochrome oxidase (that is, they are oxidase-negative).
- Among E. coli species, there are many serologically distinct O, H, and K antigens, and specific serotypes are associated with particular diseases. For example, a serotype of E. coli possessing O157 and H7 (designated O157: H7) causes a severe form of hemorrhagic colitis.
- At least five types of intestinal infections that differ in pathogenic mechanisms have been identified. Enterotoxigenic (ETEC), enteropathogenic (EPEC), enterohemorrhagic (EHEC), enteroinvasive (EIEC), and enteroaggregative (EAEC) E. coli all are basically the same organism, differing only by the acquisition of specific pathogenic traits.
- Enterohemorrhagic E. coli infection should be suspected in all patients with acute bloody diarrhea, particularly if associated with abdominal tenderness and absence of fever.
- ETEC are a common cause of traveler's diarrhea.
- Enterotoxins include a heat-stable toxin (ST) that works by causing an elevation in cellular cyclic guanosine monophosphate (cGMP) levels, whereas a heat-labile toxin (LT) causes elevated cyclic adenosine monophosphate (cAMP). [Note: LT is essentially identical to cholera toxin].
- Rifaximin is approved for the treatment of diarrhea caused by noninvasive strains of Escherichia coli in patients 12 years of age and older. Rifaximin is a nonabsorable, gastrointestinal-selective, oral antibiotic.
- Fluoroquinolones are commonly used in adults for traveler's diarrhea, but are not recommended for children.
- EHEC bind to cells in the large intestine, where they produce an exotoxin (verotoxin, or Shiga-like toxin), causing a severe form of copious, bloody diarrhea (hemorrhagic colitis) in the absence of mucosal invasion or inflammation. Serotype O157: H7 is the most common strain of E. coli that produces verotoxin.
- E. coli is the most common cause of UTI, including cystitis and pyelonephritis.
- Uncomplicated cystitis (the most commonly encountered UTI) is caused by uropathogenic strains of E. coli, characterized by P. fimbriae (an adherence factor) and, frequently, hemolysin, colicin V, and resistance to the bactericidal activity of serum complement. Complicated UTI (pyelonephritis) occurs in settings of obstructed urinary flow, which may be caused by nonuropathogenic strains.
- E. coli is a major cause of meningitis occurring within the first month of life. The K1 (capsular) antigen is particularly associated with such infections.
- EIEC strains often do not ferment lactose, and may be detected on media, such as MacConkey agar.
- EHEC, unlike most other strains of E. coli, ferment sorbitol slowly if at all, and may be detected on MacConkey sorbitol agar.
- Viridis is the Latin word for green, and most of the viridans streptococci are alpha-hemolytic, producing greenish discoloration on blood agar.
- Strep intermedius immediately assess for abscess.
- Bovis in blood, better beware cancer in bowel.
- *Streptococcus pneumoniae* is also the most common cause of otitis media (middle ear infection) in children and the most common cause of bacterial meningitis in adults. Also the most common cause of pneumonia in adults.
- Lethal factor (LF) of Bacillus anthracis is a zinc metalloprotease that inactivates protein kinase. This toxin stimulates the macrophage to release tumor necrosis factor A and interleukin-1, 3, which contribute to death in anthrax.

- Being the brightest medical student in the pediatric emergency room, you immediately recognize that this child probably has diphtheria. Realizing that you are dealing with an extremely powerful exotoxin, you quickly TELL yoUR InTErn not to 'loaf around' (Loeffler's) and tellurite medium.
- Gastroenteritis of salmonella: This localized disease (also called salmonellosis) is caused primarily by serotypes enteritidis and typhimurium (nontyphoidal salmonella).
- In typhoid, about thirty percent of patients have a faint maculopapular rash on the trunk (rose spots).
- Salmons swim. Salmonella are motile. Motile bacilli generally produce H_2S.
- Members of the genus Campylobacter are curved, spiral, or S-shaped organisms that microscopically resemble vibrios.
- C. jejuni is a cause of both traveler's diarrhea and pseudoappendicitis (symptoms simulating appendicitis without inflammation of the appendix). Bacteremia (often transient) may occur, most often in infants and the elderly. Sustained bacteremia usually reflects host compromise. Complications include septic abortion, reactive arthritis, and Guillain-Barré syndrome.
- Campylobacter can be isolated from feces using special selective media and microaerophilic conditions.
- For C. jejuni, ciprofloxacin is the drug of choice; other antibiotics are also effective.
- Shigella species cause shigellosis (bacillary dysentery) a human intestinal disease that occurs most commonly among young children. Shigellae are nonmotile, unencapsulated, and Lac. Most strains do not produce gas in a mixed acid fermentation of glucose.
- The forty serotypes of Shigella are organized into four groups (A, B, C, and D) based on the serologic relatedness of their polysaccharide O antigens. Group D (S. sonnei) is the serogroup found most commonly in the United States.
- Shigellae invade and destroy the mucosa of the large intestine. Infection rarely penetrates to deeper layers of the intestine, and does not lead to Shigella bacteremia.
- Shigellae cause classic bacillary dysentery, characterized by diarrhea with blood, mucus, and painful abdominal cramping.
- During acute illness, organisms can be cultured from stools using differential, selective Hektoen agar or other media specific for intestinal pathogens.
- The growth of many Vibrio strains either requires or is stimulated by NaCl. Pathogenic vibrios include: 1. V. cholerae, serogroup O1 strains that are associated with epidemic cholera; 2. Non-O1 V. cholerae and related strains that cause sporadic cases of cholera-like and other illnesses; and 3. V. parahaemolyticus and other halophilic vibrios, which cause gastroenteritis and extraintestinal infections.
- The A subunit of Vibrio toxin has two components: A2, which facilitates penetration of the cell membrane, and A1, an ADP-ribosyl transferase that ADP-ribosylates the membrane-bound G_s protein. G_s protein activates adenylate cyclase, which produces elevated levels of intracellular cAMP. This, in turn, causes an outflowing of ions and water to the lumen of the intestine.
- V. cholerae grows on standard media such as blood and MacConkey agars. Thiosulfate citrate bile salts sucrose (TCBS) medium can enhance isolation. The organism is oxidase-positive (Volatile Pressed Capsules Hide Nasty and Mean Looks), but further biochemical testing is necessary for specific identification of V. cholerae.
- Bacteremia is associated with high mortality, especially when caused by V. vulnificus.
- The genus Yersinia includes three species of medical importance: Y. enterocolitica and Y. pseudotuberculosis, both potential pathogens of the GI tract that are discussed in this chapter, and Y. pestis, the etiologic agent of bubonic plague.
- Y. enterocolitica and Y. pseudotuberculosis are both motile when grown at 25°C but not at 37°C. Multiple serotypes of both strains exist, and the V and W antigens are virulence factors.
- Yersinia can be cultured from appropriate specimens on MacConkey or cefsulodin-irgasan-novobiocin (CIN, a medium selective for Yersinia) agars.
- Members of the genus Helicobacter are curved or spiral organisms. They have a rapid, corkscrew motility resulting from multiple polar flagella.
- Klebsiellae are large, nonmotile bacilli that possess a luxurious capsule. They are Lac^+. K. pneumoniae and K. oxytoca cause necrotizing lobar pneumonia in individuals compromised by alcoholism, diabetes, or chronic

obstructive pulmonary disease. K. pneumoniae also causes urinary tract infections and bacteremia, particularly in hospitalized patients.

- Serratia are motile and ferment lactose slowly, if at all. The species of Serratia that most frequently causes human infection is S. marcescens. Serratia can cause extraintestinal infections such as those of the lower respiratory and urinary tracts, especially among hospitalized patients.
- Proteus species are relatively common causes of uncomplicated as well as nosocomial UTIs. Other extraintestinal infections, such as wound infections, pneumonias, and septicemias, are associated with compromised patients. Proteus organisms produce urease → catalyzes the hydrolysis of urea to ammonia → resulting alkaline environment promotes the precipitation of struvite stones containing insoluble phosphates of magnesium and phosphate.
- The obligate anerobic genus, Clostridium, consists of gram-positive, spore-forming rods that are associated with soft tissue and skin infections (for example, cellulitis and fasciitis), and antibiotic-associated colitis and diarrhea.
- Clinically significant species of Clostridium include C. perfringens, which causes histotoxic (tissue destructive) infections (myonecrosis) and food poisoning; C. difficile, which causes pseudomembranous colitis associated with antibiotic use; C. tetani, which causes tetanus (lockjaw) and C. botulinum, which causes botulism.
- Clostridia grow on enriched media in the presence of a reducing agent such as cysteine or thioglycollate (to maintain a low oxidation-reduction potential) or in an O_2-free, gaseous atmosphere provided by an air-evacuated glove box, sealed jar, or other device.
- The majority of infections resulting in necrosis of muscle are due to Clostridium species (gas gangrene) and group A streptococcus.
- Increasing pain at the site of prior injury or surgery, together with signs of systemic toxicity and gas in the soft tissue, support the diagnosis of gas gangrene
- Clostridial infections usually involve a mixture of species; therefore, the use of broad-spectrum antibiotics is appropriate.
- C. botulinum causes botulism, which occurs in several clinical forms. Botulism is caused by the action of a neurotoxin that is one of the most potent poisons known. It causes a flaccid paralysis. Contact with the organism itself is not required; hence, the disease can be a pure intoxication.
- Tetanus toxin, called tetanospasmin, is an extremely potent toxin with A and B fragments.
- The A fragment has been shown to be a protease; it cleaves a small synaptic vesicle protein (synaptobrevin) and abolishes the flow of inhibitory neurotransmitters.
- In the early stages of the disease, the jaw muscles are affected, so that the mouth cannot open (trismus, or lockjaw).
- C. tetani has a characteristic morphology, with a long, slender rod and round, terminal spore (racquet-shaped bacillus) and characteristic swarming growth on anerobic blood agar.
- So clostridium tetani is racquet-shaped. (Something we contract when we are playing tennis!)
- C. difficile is a minor component of the normal flora of the large intestine. Pathogenic strains produce two toxic polypeptides, designated A and B. Toxin A is an enterotoxin that causes excessive fluid secretion, but also stimulates an inflammatory response, and has some cytopathic effect in tissue culture. Toxin B is a cytotoxin; in tissue culture, it disrupts protein synthesis and causes disorganization of the cytoskeleton.
- Virtually all antimicrobial drugs have been reported as predisposing to clostridial AAD and colitis. The three drugs most commonly implicated are clindamycin, ampicillin, and the cephalosporins.
- Members of the genus Bacteroides are the predominant anerobes found in the human colon. They are part of the normal flora, and only cause disease when they gain access to tissues or the blood during bowel penetration (for example, during surgery or trauma). They are, however, the most common cause of serious infections by anerobic organisms. Bacteroides are slender rods or coccobacilli. Their polysaccharide capsule is an important virulence factor, conveying resistance to phagocytosis.
- The major disease-causing Bacteroides species is B. fragilis. When released from the colon into the blood, B. fragilis multiplies rapidly, causing bacteremia. If it is introduced into the abdominal cavity, B. fragilis causes peritonitis, and/or abdominal abscesses.

- Spirochetes are long, slender, motile, flexible, undulating, gram-negative bacilli that have a characteristic corkscrew or helical shape.
- Spirochetes that are important human pathogens are confined to three genera: Treponema (T. pallidum causes syphilis), Borrelia (B. burgdorferi causes Lyme disease, B. recurrentis causes relapsing fever), and Leptospira (L. interrogans causes leptospirosis).
- The spirochete cell has a central protoplasmic cylinder bounded by a plasma membrane and a typical gram-negative cell wall. Unlike other bacilli, this cylinder is enveloped by an outer sheath composed of glycosaminoglycans.
- Members of the genus Borrelia are relatively large spirochetes that, like Treponema, have endoflagella that make them highly motile.
- Borrelia species are unusual among bacteria in that they have linear rather than circular plasmid and chromosomal DNA. Like T. pallidum, Borrelia do not appear to produce endotoxins or exotoxins.
- Endemic tick born, epidemic lice born. Organism is Borrelia burgdorferi and recurrrentis respectively.
- A most striking property of B. recurrentis is its ability to change its surface protein antigens. This ability accounts for the relapsing nature of the disease because with each relapse, a new antigenic variant arises.
- The first symptoms of relapsing fever appear three to ten days after exposure to an infected arthropod. These symptoms include an abrupt onset of high fever, accompanied by severe headache, muscle pain, and general malaise.
- L. interrogans infection causes the disease leptospirosis. The organism is a slender (lepto = slender), tightly coiled, culturable spirochete with a single, thin, axial filament, and hooked ends.
- *Staphylococcus aureus* causes abscesses, various pyogenic infections (e.g. endocarditis, septic arthritis, and osteomyelitis), food poisoning, scalded skin syndrome, and toxic shock syndrome. It is one of the most common causes of hospital-acquired pneumonia, septicemia, and surgical-wound infections. It is an important cause of skin infections, such as folliculitis, cellulitis, and impetigo. *Staphylococcus epidermidis* can cause endocarditis and prosthetic joint infections. *Staphylococcus saprophyticus* causes urinary tract infections. Kawasaki syndrome is a disease of unknown etiology that may be caused by certain strains of *S. aureus.*
- Group B streptococci (*S. agalactiae*) colonize the genital tract of some women and can cause neonatal meningitis and sepsis. They are usually bacitracin-resistant. They hydrolyze (breakdown) hippurate, an important diagnostic criterion.
- Group D streptococci include enterococci (e.g. *Enterococcus faecalis* and *Enterococcus faecium*) and nonenterococci (e.g. *S. bovis*).
- The principal alpha-hemolytic organisms are *S. pneumoniae* and the viridans group of streptococci.
- The term 'mixed anerobic infections' refers to the fact that these infections are caused by multiple bacteria, some of which are anerobes and others are facultatives. For example, peptostreptococci and viridans streptococci, both members of the oral flora, are often found in brain abscesses following dental surgery. *Peptostreptococcus magnus* and *Peptostreptococcus anaerobius* are the species frequently isolated from clinical specimens.
- The injection of a skin test dose of erythrogenic toxin (Dick test) gives a positive result in persons lacking antitoxin (i.e. susceptible persons).
- *S. bovis*, a nonenterococcal group D streptococcus, causes endocarditis, especially in patients with carcinoma of the colon. This association is so strong that patients with *S. bovis* bacteremia or endocarditis should be investigated for the presence of colonic carcinoma.
- The eukaryotic cell membrane contains sterols, whereas no prokaryote, except the wall-less Mycoplasma, has sterols in its membranes.
- Spore has a keratin-like coat made of dipicolinic acid.
- Synonyms for peptidoglycan are murein and mucopeptide.
- Teichoic acids are fibers of glycerol phosphate or ribitol phosphate and are located in the outer layer of the gram-positive cell wall and extend from it. Some polymers of glycerol teichoic acid penetrate the peptidoglycan layer and are covalently linked to the lipid in the cytoplasmic membrane, in which case they are called lipoteichoic acid.

- The cytoplasm contains several different types of granules that serve as storage areas for nutrients and stain characteristically with certain dyes. For example, volutin is a reserve of high energy stored in the form of polymerized metaphosphate. It appears as a 'metachromatic' granule, since it stains red with methylene blue dye instead of blue, as one would expect. Metachromatic granules are a characteristic feature of *Corynebacterium diphtheria.*
- Pityriasis versicolor and tinea nigra are extremely superficial fungus infections, whose primary manifestation is pigment change of the skin.
- Pityriasis versicolor (also called tinea versicolor) is a chronic superficial fungal infection which leads to hypopigmented or hyperpigmented patches on the skin. This infection is caused *by Malassezia furfur.*
- Tinea nigra is caused *by Exophiala werneckii.*
- The common dermatophytes include Microsporum, Trichophyton, and Epidermophyton.
- Three fungi that cause systemic disease in humans are *Histoplasma capsulatum, Blastomyces dermatitidis,* and *Coccidioides immitis.*
- *Cryptococcus neoformans* is a polysaccharide encapsulated yeast (not dimorphic) similar to the previous 3 fungi in that it is inhaled into the lungs and the infection is usually asymptomatic. It differs in that the major manifestation is not pneumonia but rather meningoencephalitis.
IMIDAZOLES	TRIAZOLES
Ketoconazole	Fluconazole
Miconazole	Itraconazole
Clotrimazole (KMC)	Voriconazole (FIV)
- Chitin is a polysaccharide composed of long chains of *N*-acetylglucosamine. The fungal cell wall contains other polysaccharides as well, the most important of which is β-glucan, a long polymer of D-glucose. The medical importance of β-glucan is that it is the site of action of the antifungal drug caspofungin.
- Most fungi are obligate aerobes; some are facultative anerobes; but none are obligate anerobes.
- Some fungi reproduce sexually by mating and forming sexual spores, e.g. zygospores, ascospores, and basidiospores.
- Zygospores are single large spores with thick walls; ascospores are formed in a sac called ascus; and basidiospores are formed externally on the tip of a pedestal called a basidium. The classification of these fungi is based on their sexual spores. Fungi that do not form sexual spores are termed as 'imperfect' and are classified as fungi imperfecti.
- The best-known mycotoxicosis occurs after eating *Amanita* mushrooms. These fungi produce five toxins, two of which—amanitin and phalloidin—are among the most potent hepatotoxins.
- Another mycotoxicosis, ergotism, is caused by the mold *Claviceps purpurea,* which infects grains and produces alkaloids (e.g. ergotamine and lysergic acid diethylamide [LSD]) that cause pronounced vascular and neurologic effects.
- There are four approaches to the laboratory diagnosis of fungal diseases:
  - Direct microscopic examination
  - Culture of the organism
  - DNA probe tests, and
  - Serologic tests.
- Calcofluor white is a fluorescent dye that binds to fungal cell walls and is useful in the identification of fungi in tissue specimens. Methenamine-silver stain is also useful in the microscopic diagnosis of fungi in tissue.
- Trichophyton tonsurans is the most common cause of outbreaks of tinea capitis in children and is the main cause of endothrix (inside the hair) infections. Trichophyton rubrum is also a very common cause of tinea capitis. Trichophyton schoenleinii is the cause of favus, a form of tinea capitis in which crusts are seen on the scalp.
- Tinea capitis lesions caused by *Microsporum* species can be detected by seeing fluorescence when the lesions are exposed to ultraviolet light from a Wood's lamp.
- Tinea versicolor (pityriasis versicolor), a superficial skin infection of cosmetic importance only, is caused by *Malassezia furfur.*

- Tinea nigra is an infection of the keratinized layers of the skin. It appears as a brownish spot caused by the melanin-like pigment in the hyphae. The causative organism, *Cladosporium werneckii,* is found in the soil and transmitted during injury.
- Sporotrichosis occurs most often in gardeners, especially those who prune roses, because they may be stuck by a rose thorn. In the clinical laboratory, round or cigar-shaped budding yeasts are seen in tissue specimens. In culture, hyphae occur bearing oval conidia in clusters at the tip of slender conidiophores (resembling a daisy). The drug of choice for skin lesions is itraconazole.
- Chromomycosis is a slowly progressive granulomatous infection that is caused by several soil fungi (*Fonsecaea, Phialophora, Cladosporium,* etc.) when introduced into the skin through trauma. These fungi are collectively called dematiaceous fungi, so named because their conidia or hyphae are dark-colored, either gray or black.
- *Mycetoma*: Soil organisms (*Petriellidium, Madurella*) enter through wounds on the feet, hands, or back and cause abscesses, with pus discharged through sinuses. The pus contains compact-colored granules. Actinomycetes such as *Nocardia* can cause similar lesions (actinomycotic mycetoma).
- *Coccidioides immitis*: About 50% have changes in the lungs (infiltrates, adenopathy, or effusions) as seen on chest X-ray, and 10% develop erythema nodosum or arthralgias. This syndrome is called 'valley fever' (in the San Joaquin Valley of California) or 'desert rheumatism' (in Arizona); it tends to subside spontaneously. If meningitis occurs, fluconazole is the drug of choice.
- The yeasts of Histoplasma survive within the phagolysosome of the macrophage by producing alkaline substances, such as bicarbonate and ammonia, that raise the pH and thereby inactivate the degradative enzymes of the phagolysosome.
- In AIDS patients, ulcerated lesions on the tongue are typical of disseminated histoplasmosis. In immunocompetent people, EN can occur. EN is a sign that cell-mediated immunity is active and the organism will probably be contained.
- Two serologic tests are useful for diagnosis: complement fixation (CF) and immunodiffusion (ID). An antibody titer of 1: 32 in the CF test with yeast phase antigens is considered to be diagnostic. However, cross-reactions with other fungi, especially *Blastomyces,* occur. CF titers fall when the disease becomes inactive and there is a rise in disseminated disease. The ID test detects precipitating antibodies (precipitins) by forming two bands, M and H, in an agar-gel diffusion assay. The ID test is more specific but less sensitive than the CF test.
- *B. dermatitidis* is a dimorphic fungus that exists as a mold in soil and as a yeast in tissue. The yeast is round with a doubly refractive wall and a single broad-based bud. Note that this organism forms a broad-based bud, whereas *Cryptococcus neoformans* is a yeast that forms a narrow-based bud.
- *P. brasiliensis* is a dimorphic fungus that exists as a mold in soil and as a yeast in tissue. The yeast is thick-walled with multiple buds, in contrast to *B. dermatitidis,* which has a single bud.
- *C. albicans* is an oval yeast with a single bud.
- In exudates or tissues, budding yeasts and pseudohyphae appear gram-positive and can be visualized using calcofluor-white staining. In culture, typical yeast colonies are formed that resemble large staphylococcal colonies. Germ tubes form in serum at 37°C, which serves to distinguish *C. albicans* from most other *Candida* species. Chlamydospores are typically formed by *C. albicans* but not by other species of *Candida.* Serologic testing is rarely helpful.
- The drug of choice for oropharyngeal or esophageal thrush is fluconazole. Caspofungin or micafungin can also be used for esophageal candidiasis.
- *Cryptococcus*: Serologic tests can be done for both antibody and antigen. In infected spinal fluid, capsular antigen occurs in high titer and can be detected by the latex particle agglutination test. This test is called the cryptococcal antigen test, often abbreviated as 'crag'.
- *Aspergillus* species exist only as molds; they are not dimorphic. They have septate hyphae that form V-shaped (dichotomous) branches. The walls are more or less parallel, in contrast to *Mucor* and *Rhizopus* walls, which are irregular. The conidia of *Aspergillus* form radiating chains, in contrast to those of *Mucor* and *Rhizopus,* which are enclosed within a sporangium.
- *A. fumigatus* can colonize and later invade abraded skin, wounds, burns, the cornea, the external ear, or paranasal sinuses. It is the most common cause of fungal sinusitis.

- *Aspergillus flavus* growing on cereals or nuts produces aflatoxins that may be carcinogenic or acutely toxic.
- Mucormycosis (zygomycosis, phycomycosis) is a disease caused by saprophytic molds (e.g. *Mucor, Rhizopus,* and *Absidia*) found widely in the environment. They are not dimorphic.
- One species, *Rhizopus oryzae,* causes about 60% of the cases of mucormycosis.
- In biopsy specimens, organisms are seen microscopically as nonseptate hyphae with broad, irregular walls and branches that form more or less at right angles. Cultures show colonies with spores contained within a sporangium.

  Lecture
- Mnemonic for dimorphic fungi is '***Body Heat Changes Shape***': Blastomyces, Histoplasma, Coccidioides and Sporothrix.
- Mold in Cold, Yeast in Beast.
- ***All the Bs: Broad-based Budding Blastomyces.***
- The DNA is always a single molecule; the RNA can exist either as a single molecule or in several pieces. For example, both influenza virus and rotavirus have a segmented RNA genome.
- The nucleic acid is surrounded by a protein coat called **capsid**, made up of subunits called capsomers. Each capsomer, consisting of one or several proteins, can be seen in the electron microscope as a spherical particle, sometimes with a central hole.
- All human viruses that have a helical nucleocapsid are enclosed by an outer membrane called an **envelope**, i.e. there are no naked helical viruses.
- The advantage of building the virus particle from identical protein subunits is twofold: (1) it reduces the need for genetic information and (2) it promotes self-assembly; i.e. no enzyme or energy is required. In fact, functional virus particles have been assembled in the test tube by combining the purified nucleic acid with the purified proteins in the absence of cells, energy source, and enzymes.
- If a virus has an envelope, then a matrix protein that mediates the interaction between the capsid proteins and the envelope proteins is present.
- Viruses known to produce superantigens include two members of the herpesvirus family, namely, Epstein-Barr virus and cytomegalovirus, and the retrovirus mouse mammary tumor virus.
- The envelope of most viruses is derived from the cell's outer membrane, with the notable exception of herpesviruses that derive their envelope from the cell's nuclear membrane.
- Members of the herpesvirus family, such as herpes simplex virus and cytomegalovirus, have a prominent, well-characterized tegument.
- **Viroids** consist solely of a single molecule of circular RNA without a protein coat or envelope.
- **Retrovirus** is diploid.
- Rabies virus binds to the acetylcholine receptor, Epstein-Barr virus binds to a complement receptor, vaccinia virus binds to the receptor for epidermal growth factor, and rhinovirus binds to the integrin ICAM-1.
- **The genome of all DNA viruses consists of double-stranded DNA, except for the parvoviruses, which have a single-stranded DNA genome.**
- All DNA viruses encode their own DNA polymerase that replicates the genome. They do not use the host cell DNA polymerase.
- Most RNA viruses undergo their entire replicative cycle in the cytoplasm. The two principal exceptions are retroviruses and influenza viruses, both of which have an important replicative step in the nucleus.
- **The genome of all RNA viruses consists of single-stranded RNA, except for members of the reovirus family, which have a double-stranded RNA genome.** Rotavirus is the important human pathogen in the reovirus family.
- ***Inclusion bodies*** are aggregates of virions in specific locations in the cell that are useful for laboratory diagnosis. Two important examples are ***Negri bodies*** in the cytoplasm of rabies virus-infected cells and ***owl's eye inclusions*** in the nucleus of cytomegalovirus-infected cells.
- One type of immunopathogenesis is the ***killing of virus-infected cell by the attack of cytotoxic T cells*** that recognize viral antigens on the cell surface. Damage to the liver caused by hepatitis viruses occurs by this

mechanism. Another is the ***formation of virus-antibody complexes that are deposited in tissues.*** Arthritis associated with parvovirus B19 or rubella virus infection occurs by this mechanism.

- In CMV-infected cells, assembly of the MHC class I–viral peptide complex is unstable, so viral antigens are not displayed on the cell surface and killing by cytotoxic T cells does not occur.
- In immunocompetent adults, CMV can cause **heterophil-negative mononucleosis,** which is characterized by fever, lethargy, and the presence of abnormal lymphocytes in peripheral blood smears. Systemic CMV infections, especially pneumonitis and hepatitis, occur in a high proportion of immunosuppressed patients, e.g. those with renal and bone marrow transplants. In AIDS patients, CMV commonly infects the intestinal tract and causes intractable colitis. CMV also causes retinitis in AIDS patients, which can lead to blindness.
- CMV antigenemia can be measured by detecting pp65 within blood leukocytes using an immunofluorescence assay. pp65 is a protein located in the nucleocapsid of CMV and can be identified within infected leukocytes using fluorescein-labeled monoclonal antibody specific for pp65.
- EBV causes infectious mononucleosis. It is associated with Burkitt's lymphoma, other B-cell lymphomas, and nasopharyngeal carcinoma. EBV is also associated with hairy leukoplakia, a whitish, nonmalignant lesion on the tongue seen especially in AIDS patients.
- EBV is structurally and morphologically identical to other herpesviruses but is antigenically different. The most important antigen is the **viral capsid antigen** (VCA), because it is used most often in diagnostic tests.
- The early antigens (EA), which are produced prior to viral DNA synthesis, and nuclear antigen (EBNA), which is located in the nucleus bound to chromosomes, are sometimes diagnostically helpful as well.
- EBV enters B lymphocytes at the site of the receptor for the C3 component of complement.
- EBV is transmitted primarily by the exchange of saliva, e.g. during kissing. The saliva of people with a reactivation of a latent infection as well as people with an active infection can serve as a source of the virus. In contrast to CMV, blood transmission of EBV is very rare.
- Kindly note this, it is very important: The frequency of clinically apparent infectious mononucleosis, however, is highest in those who are exposed to the virus later in life, e.g. college students.
- Infectious mononucleosis is characterized primarily by fever, sore throat, lymphadenopathy, and splenomegaly. Anorexia and lethargy are prominent. Hepatitis is frequent; encephalitis occurs in some patients. Spontaneous recovery usually occurs in 2–3 weeks. Splenic rupture, associated with contact sports, such as football, is a feared but rare complication of the splenomegaly.
- KS in AIDS patients is a malignancy of vascular endothelial cells that contains many spindle-shaped cells and erythrocytes. The lesions are dark purple, flat to nodular, and often appear at multiple sites, such as the skin, oral cavity, and soles (but not the palms).
- An EBV envelope glycoprotein binds to CD21 (CR2), the receptor for the C3d component of complement, present on B cells.
- The gene products include EBNA1, which binds the EBV genome to chromosomes, mediating episomal persistence and maintenance, and EBNA2 and latent membrane protein 1 (LMP1), which drive B-cell activation and proliferation.
- LMP1 appears to act by binding to TNF receptor–associated factors, and activates signalling pathways that mimic B-cell activation by CD40, which is involved in normal B-cell responses.
- The virulence of the H5N1 strain is significantly greater than the H1N1 and H3N2 strains that have been causing disease in humans for many years. This is attributed to two features of the H5N1 strain, namely relative resistance to interferon and increased induction of cytokines, especially TNF. The increase in cytokines is thought to mediate the pathogenesis of the pneumonia and acute respiratory distress syndrome (ARDS) seen in H5N1 infection.
- 1968-H3N2
- 1918-H5N1 resemblance
- 1997-H5N1
- Severe myalgias (muscle pains) coupled with respiratory tract symptoms are typical of influenza.
- This virus causes measles, a disease characterized by a maculopapular rash. It occurs primarily in childhood.

- In malnourished children, especially those in developing countries, measles is a much more serious disease than in well-nourished children. Vitamin A deficiency is especially important in this regard, and supplementation of this vitamin greatly reduces the severity of measles.
- After infecting the cells lining the upper respiratory tract, the virus enters the blood and infects reticuloendothelial cells, where it replicates again. It then spreads via the blood to the skin. The **rash** is caused primarily by cytotoxic T cells attacking the measles virus-infected vascular endothelial cells in the skin.
- Infection with measles virus can **transiently depress cell-mediated immunity** against other intracellular microorganisms, such as *Mycobacterium tuberculosis,* leading to a loss of PPD skin test reactivity, reactivation of dormant organisms, and clinical disease. The proposed mechanism for this unusual finding is that when measles virus binds to its receptor (called CD46) on the surface of human macrophages, the production of IL-12, which is necessary for cell-mediated immunity to occur, is suppressed.
- Two cell-surface receptors have been identified for the virus: CD46, a complement-regulatory protein that inactivates C3 convertases, and signaling lymphocytic activation molecule (SLAM), a molecule involved in T-cell activation.
- The lymphoid organs typically have marked follicular hyperplasia, large germinal centers, and randomly distributed multinucleate giant cells, called Warthin-Finkeldey cells, which have eosinophilic nuclear and cytoplasmic inclusion bodies. These are pathognomonic of measles and are also found in the lung and sputum.
- This virus causes mumps, a disease characterized by parotid gland swelling. It occurs primarily in childhood.
- There is a characteristic increase in parotid pain when drinking citrus juices.
- Mumps virus, coxsackievirus, and echovirus are the three most frequent causes of viral (aseptic) meningitis. The widespread use of the vaccine in the United States has led to a marked decrease in the incidence of mumps meningitis.
- Respiratory syncytial virus (RSV) is the most important cause of pneumonia and bronchiolitis in infants. It is also an important cause of otitis media in children and of pneumonia in the elderly and in patients with chronic cardiopulmonary diseases.
- RSV infection in **infants is more severe** and more often involves the lower respiratory tract than in older children and adults. The infection is localized to the respiratory tract; viremia does not occur.
- The severe disease in infants may have an **immunopathogenic** mechanism. Maternal antibody passed to the infant may react with the virus, form immune complexes, and damage the respiratory tract cells. Trials with a killed vaccine resulted in more severe disease, an unexpected finding that supports such a mechanism.
- *Para-influenza*: These viruses cause croup (acute laryngotracheobronchitis), laryngitis, bronchiolitis, and pneumonia in children and a disease resembling the common cold in adults.
- There are four types, which are distinguished by antigenicity, cytopathic effect, and pathogenicity. Parainfluenza viruses 1 and 2 are **major causes of croup**. Parainfluenza virus 3 is the most common parainfluenzavirus isolated from children with lower respiratory tract infection in the United States. Parainfluenza virus 4 rarely causes disease, except for the common cold.
- In 1967, the World Health Organization embarked on a vaccination campaign that led to the eradication of smallpox. The last naturally occurring case was in Somalia in 1977.
- After an incubation period of 7–14 days, there is a sudden onset of prodromal symptoms, such as fever and malaise. This is followed by the rash, which is worse on the face and extremities than on the trunk (i.e. it has a centrifugal distribution). The rash evolves through stages from macules to papules, vesicles, pustules, and, finally, crusts in 2–3 weeks.
- The disease was eradicated by global use of the **vaccine**, which contains live, attenuated **vaccinia virus**. The success of the vaccine is dependent upon five critical factors: (1) smallpox virus has a single, stable serotype; (2) there is no animal reservoir, and humans are the only hosts; (3) the antibody response is prompt; therefore, exposed persons can be protected; (4) the disease is easily recognized clinically; therefore, exposed persons can be immunized promptly; and (5) there is no carrier state or subclinical infection.
- In the past, methisazone was used to treat the complications of vaccination and could be useful again.
- Human papillomavirus (HPV) causes papillomas, which are benign tumors of squamous cells, e.g. warts on the skin. Some HPV types, especially types 16 and 18, cause **carcinoma of the cervix and penis.**

- Skin warts are caused primarily by HPV-1 through HPV-4, whereas genital warts are usually caused by HPV-6 and HPV-11.
- Occult premalignant lesions of the cervix and penis can be revealed by applying acetic acid to the tissue.
- Parvovirus B19 causes erythema infectiosum (slapped cheek syndrome, fifth disease), aplastic anemia (especially in patients with sickle-cell anemia), and fetal infections, including hydrops fetalis.
- B19 virus is transmitted primarily by the respiratory route; transplacental transmission also occurs. Blood donated for transfusions also can transmit the virus.
- Erythema infectiosum (slapped cheek syndrome, fifth disease), measles, rubella, scarlet fever, and roseola are macular or maculopapular rash diseases of childhood.
- Parvovirus B19 infection in adults, especially women, can cause arthritis mainly involving the small joints of the hands and feet bilaterally. It resembles rheumatoid arthritis. Other viral infections that cause an immune-complex-related arthritis include hepatitis B and rubella.
- Paramyxoviruses are composed of **one piece** of single-stranded RNA, a helical nucleocapsid, and an outer lipoprotein envelope. The virion contains an RNA-dependent **RNA polymerase**, which transcribes the **negative-polarity** genome into mRNA. The genome is, therefore, not infectious. The envelope is covered with spikes, which contain hemagglutinin, neuraminidase, or a fusion protein that causes cell fusion and, in some cases, hemolysis.
- Infection with measles virus can **transiently depress cell-mediated immunity** against other intracellular microorganisms, such as *Mycobacterium tuberculosis,* leading to a loss of PPD skin test reactivity, reactivation of dormant organisms, and clinical disease. The proposed mechanism for this unusual finding is that when measles virus binds to its receptor (called CD46) on the surface of human macrophages, the production of IL-12, which is necessary for cell-mediated immunity to occur, is suppressed.
- Most diagnoses are made on clinical grounds, but the virus can be isolated in cell culture; a rise in antibody titer of greater than fourfold can be used to diagnose difficult cases.
- *Mumps virus*: The internal nucleocapsid protein is the S (soluble) antigen detected in the complement fixation test used for diagnosis.
- The virus can be isolated in cell culture from saliva, spinal fluid, or urine. In addition, a fourfold rise in antibody titer in either the hemagglutination inhibition or the CF test is diagnostic.
- A single CF test that assays both the S and the V (viral) antigens can also be used. Because antibody to S antigen appears early and is shortlived, it indicates current infection. If only V antibody is found, the patient has had mumps in the past.
- Mumps virus, coxsackievirus, and echovirus are the three most frequent causes of viral (aseptic) meningitis.
- Respiratory syncytial virus (RSV) is the most important cause of pneumonia and bronchiolitis in infants. It is also an important cause of otitis media in children and of pneumonia in the elderly and in patients with chronic cardiopulmonary diseases.
- An enzyme immunoassay ('rapid antigen test') that detects the presence of RSV antigens in respiratory secretions is commonly used. The presence of the virus can be detected by immunofluorescence on smears of respiratory epithelium or by isolation in cell culture. The cytopathic effect in cell culture is characterized by the formation of multinucleated giant cells. A rise in antibody titer of at least 4-fold is also diagnostic. A reverse transcriptase polymerase chain reaction (RRT-PCR) test is also available.
- Parainfluenza viruses 1 and 2 are **major causes of croup**. Parainfluenza virus 3 is the most common parainfluenzavirus isolated from children with lower respiratory tract infection in the United States. Parainfluenza virus 4 rarely causes disease, except for the common cold.
- Most infections are diagnosed clinically. The diagnosis can be made in the laboratory either by isolating the virus in cell culture or by observing a fourfold or greater rise in antibody titer.
- Coronaviruses are an important cause of the common cold, probably second only to rhinoviruses in frequency.
- Coronaviruses have a nonsegmented, single-stranded, positive-polarity RNA genome. They are enveloped viruses with a helical nucleocapsid.
- In the electron microscope, prominent club-shaped spikes in the form of a 'corona' (halo) can be seen. There are two serotypes called 229E and OC43.

- The virus is assembled and obtains its envelope from the endoplasmic reticulum, not from the plasma membrane. Replication occurs in the cytoplasm.
- The horseshoe bat appears to be the natural reservoir for CoV-SARS, with the civet cat serving as an intermediate host.
- Pneumonia caused by SARS coronavirus is characterized by diffuse edema resulting in hypoxia.
- SARS is a severe atypical pneumonia characterized by a fever of at least 38°C, nonproductive cough, dyspnea, and hypoxia. Chills, rigors, malaise, and headache commonly occur, but sore throat and rhinorrhea are uncommon. Chest x-ray reveals interstitial "ground-glass" infiltrates that do not cavitate. Leukopenia and thrombocytopenia are seen. The incubation period for SARS ranges from 2 to 10 days, with a mean of 5 days.
- Rubella Virus: This virus causes rubella (German measles) and congenital rubella syndrome. Congenital rubella syndrome is characterized by **congenital malformations.**
- Rubella virus is a member of the togavirus family.
- It is composed of one piece of single-stranded RNA, an **icosahedral** nucleocapsid, and a lipoprotein **envelope.** However, unlike the paramyxoviruses, such as measles and mumps viruses, it has a positive-strand RNA and therefore has no virion polymerase.
- Rubella is a milder, shorter disease than measles. After an incubation period of 14–21 days, a brief prodromal period with fever and malaise is followed by a maculopapular rash, which starts on the face and progresses downward to involve the extremities. Posterior auricular lymphadenopathy is characteristic. The rash typically lasts 3 days. When rubella occurs in adults, especially women, polyarthritis caused by immune complexes often occurs.
- Rubella virus can be grown in cell culture, but it produces little cytopathic effect (CPE). It is therefore usually identified by its ability to interfere with echovirus CPE.
- Rabies virus is the only medically important member of the rhabdovirus family. It has a **single-stranded RNA** enclosed within a **bullet-shaped** capsid surrounded by a lipoprotein **envelope**· Because the genome RNA has **negative polarity**, the virion contains an RNA-dependent **RNA polymerase**. Rabies virus has a single antigenic type. The antigenicity resides in the envelope glycoprotein spikes.
- Rabies virus attaches to the **acetylcholine receptor** on the cell surface.
- Rabies in humans can be diagnosed by fluorescent-antibody staining of a biopsy specimen, usually taken from the skin of the neck at the hairline; by isolation of the virus from sources, such as saliva, spinal fluid, and brain tissue; or by a rise in titer of antibody to the virus. Negri bodies can be demonstrated in corneal scrapings and in autopsy specimens of the brain.
- In the United States, the **rabies vaccine** contains inactivated virus grown in human diploid cells (HDCV). (Vaccine grown in monkey lung cells or chick embryo cells is also available.) In other countries, the duck embryo vaccine or various nerve tissue vaccines are available as well.
- Five doses of HDCV are given (on days 0, 3, 7, 14, and 28), but RIG is given only once with the first dose of HDCV (at a different site).
- The vaccine for immunization of dogs and cats consists of inactivated rabies virus. The first immunization is usually given at 3 months of age, with booster doses given either annually or at 3-year intervals. In the United States, an alternative vaccine used in dogs and cats contains live canarypox virus genetically engineered to contain the gene for the envelope protein of rabies virus.
- Human T-cell lymphotropic virus-1 (HTLV) causes two distinctly different diseases: a cancer called adult T-cell leukemia/lymphoma and a neurologic disease called HTLV-associated myelopathy (also known as tropical spastic paraparesis or chronic progressive myelopathy). HTLV-2 also appears to cause these diseases, but the association is less clearly documented.
- The genes in the HTLV genome whose functions have been clearly identified are the three structural genes common to all retroviruses, namely, *gag*, *pol*, and *env*, plus two regulatory genes, *tax* and *rex*. In general, HTLV genes and proteins are similar to those of HIV in size and function, but the genes differ in base sequence and, therefore, the proteins differ in amino acid sequence (and antigenicity). For example, p24 is the major nucleocapsid protein in both HTLV and HIV, but they differ antigenically. The virions of both HTLV and HIV

contain a reverse transcriptase, integrase, and protease. The envelope proteins of HTLV are gp46 and gp21, whereas those of HIV are gp120 and gp41.

- The proteins encoded by the *tax* and *rex* genes play the same functional roles as those encoded by the HIV regulatory genes, *tat* and *rev*. The Tax protein is a transcriptional activator, and the Rex protein governs the processing of viral mRNA and its export from the nucleus to the cytoplasm. Tax protein is required for malignant transformation of T cells.
- The Tax protein activates the synthesis of IL-2 (which is T-cell growth factor) and of the IL-2 receptor. IL-2 promotes rapid T-cell growth and eventually malignant transformation of the T cell.
- ATL is characterized by lymphadenopathy, hepatosplenomegaly, lytic bone lesions, and skin lesions. These features are caused by proliferating T cells infiltrating these organs. In the blood, the malignant T cells have a distinct 'flower-shaped' nucleus.
- Infection with HTLV is determined by detecting antibodies against the virus in the patient's serum using the ELISA test. The Western blot assay is used to confirm a positive ELISA result. PCR assay can detect the presence of HTLV RNA or DNA within the infected cells. Isolation of HTLV in cell culture from the patient's specimens is not done.
- Picornaviruses are small (20–30 nm) **nonenveloped** viruses composed of an **icosahedral nucleocapsid** and a **single-stranded** RNA genome. The genome RNA has positive polarity, i.e. on entering the cell, it functions as the viral mRNA. The genome RNA is unusual because it has a protein on the 5′ end that serves as a primer for transcription by RNA polymerase. Picornaviruses replicate in the cytoplasm of cells. They are not inactivated by lipid solvents, such as ether, because they do not have an envelope.
- The picornavirus family includes two groups of medical importance: the **enteroviruses** and the **rhinoviruses**. Among the major enteroviruses are poliovirus, coxsackieviruses, echoviruses, and hepatitis A virus. Enteroviruses infect primarily the enteric tract, whereas rhinoviruses are found in the nose and throat (rhino = nose.
- Human immunodeficiency virus (HIV) is the cause of acquired immunodeficiency syndrome (AIDS). Formerly known as human T-lymphotropic virus type 3 (HTLV-III), lymphadenopathy-associated virus (LAV), and AIDS-related virus (ARV).
- *Vif*: Enhances infectivity by inhibiting the action of APOBEC3G, an enzyme that causes hypermutation in retroviral DNA.
- *Vpr*: Transports viral core from cytoplasm into nucleus in nondividing cells.
- *Vpu*: Enhances virion release from cell.
- On the basis of differences in the base sequence of the gene that encodes gp120, HIV has been subdivided into subtypes (**clades**) A through I.
- Subtype B preferentially infects mononuclear cells and appears to be passed readily during anal sex, whereas subtype E preferentially infects female genital tract cells and appears to be passed readily during vaginal sex.
- Reverse transcriptase is a bifunctional enzyme; it also has ribonuclease H activity. Ribonuclease H degrades RNA when it is in the form of an RNA-DNA hybrid molecule.
- There is evidence that chimpanzees living in West Africa were the source of HIV-1.
- Simian immunodeficiency virus (SIV) was isolated from monkeys with an AIDS-like illness. Antibodies in some African women cross-react with SIV. The proteins of SIV resemble those of HIV-2 more closely than they resemble those of the original HIV isolates.
- One of the best characterized mutations is the delta-32 mutation in which 32 base pairs are deleted from the CCR5 gene.
- 1981: AIDS was first reported.
- AIDS is the fourth leading cause of death worldwide. (Ischemic heart disease, cerebrovascular disease, and acute lower respiratory disease are ranked first, second, and third, respectively.)
- Another explanation why some HIV-infected individuals are long-term 'nonprogressors' may lie in their ability to produce large amounts of α-Defensins. α-Defensins are a family of positively charged peptides with antibacterial activity. In 2002, they were shown to also have antiviral activity. They interfere with HIV binding to the CXCR4 receptor and block entry of the virus into the cell.

- As far as the prognosis is concerned, a patient with more than 10,000 copies of viral RNA/mL of plasma is significantly more likely to progress to AIDS than a patient with fewer than 10,000 copies.
- A syndrome called AIDS-related complex (ARC) can occur during the latent period. The most frequent manifestations are persistent fevers, fatigue, weight loss, and lymphadenopathy. ARC often progresses to AIDS.
- HBV is a member of the hepadnavirus family. It is a 42-nm **enveloped** virion, with an icosahedral nucleocapsid core containing a **partially double-stranded circular** DNA genome.
- HCV is a member of the flavivirus family. It is an enveloped virion containing a genome of single-stranded, positive-polarity RNA. It has no virion polymerase.
- In the United States, about 1% of blood donors have antibody to HCV. Commercially prepared immune globulin preparations are generally very safe, but several instances of the transmission of HCV have occurred. **This is the only example of an infectious disease transmitted by immune globulins**.
- Cirrhosis resulting from chronic HCV infection is the most common indication for liver transplantation.
- HCV infection also leads to significant autoimmune reactions, including vasculitis, arthralgias, purpura, and membranoproliferative glomerulonephritis. **HCV is the main cause of essential mixed cryoglobulinemia.** The cryoprecipitates often are composed of HCV antigens and antibodies.
- HDV is an enveloped virus with an RNA genome that is a single-stranded, negative-polarity, covalently closed circle. The RNA genome of HDV is very small and encodes only one protein, the internal core protein called **delta antigen**.
- HEV is a nonenveloped, single-stranded RNA virus tentatively classified as a member of the calicivirus family. Taxonomists have recently placed hepatitis E virus into its own genus called hepevirus. Clinically the disease resembles hepatitis A, with the exception of a high mortality rate in pregnant women.
- In 1996, hepatitis G virus (HGV) was isolated from patients with posttransfusion hepatitis. HGV is a member of the flavivirus family, as is HCV. Patients coinfected with HIV and HGV have a lower mortality rate and have less HIV in their blood than those infected with HIV alone. It is hypothesized that HGV may interfere with the replication of HIV. (HGV is also known as GB virus C.)
- A new group of viruses called **roboviruses** has recently emerged. The term 'robo' refers to the fact that these viruses are *ro*dent-*bo*rne, that is, they are transmitted directly from rodents to humans without an arthropod vector. Transmission occurs when dried rodent excrement is inhaled into the human lung, as when sweeping the floor of a cabin. Two roboviruses cause a respiratory distress syndrome that is often fatal: Sin Nombre virus (a Hantavirus) and Whitewater Arroyo virus (an arenavirus).
- Alphaviruses include Chikungunya, Mayaro, O'Nyong-Nyong, Ross River, Semliki Forest viruses, Eastern equine encephalitis virus, Western equine encephalitis virus.
- Flaviviruses include St. Louis encephalitis virus, Murray Valley encephalitis, Japanese encephalitis, dengue virus, Kyasanur Forest, yellow fever virus, Omsk hemorrhagic fever, Powassan encephalitis viruses, and West Nile viruses.
- Bunyaviruses include California encephalitis virus, Bunyamwera complex of viruses and Oropouche virus.
- Reo virus includes Colorado tick fever virus.
- Togaviruses are characterized by an icosahedral nucleocapsid surrounded by an envelope and a single-stranded, positive-polarity RNA genome. They are 70 nm in diameter, in contrast to the flaviviruses, which are 40–50 nm in diameter. Togaviruses are divided into two families, alphaviruses and rubiviruses. The only rubivirus is rubella virus.
- Bunyaviruses have a helical nucleocapsid surrounded by an envelope and a genome consisting of three segments of negative-polarity RNA that are hydrogen-bonded together.
- The diseases caused by arboviruses range in severity from mild to rapidly fatal. The clinical picture usually fits one of the three categories: (1) **encephalitis**; (2) **hemorrhagic fever**; or (3) fever with myalgias, arthralgias, and nonhemorrhagic rash.
- Eastern equine encephalitis (EEE) virus causes the **most severe** disease and is associated with the highest fatality rate (approximately 50%). In its natural habitat, the virus is transmitted primarily by the swamp **mosquito,** *Culiseta,* among the small wild birds of the Atlantic and Gulf Coast states. Species of *Aedes* mosquitoes are suspected of carrying the virus from its **wild-bird reservoir** to the principal **dead-end hosts, horses** and **humans.**

- Western equine encephalitis (WEE) virus causes disease more frequently than does EEE virus, but the illness is less severe. Inapparent infections outnumber the apparent by at least 100:1. The virus is transmitted primarily by *Culex* **mosquitoes** among the **wild-bird** population of the western states, especially in areas with irrigated farmland.
- Colorado tick fever (CTF) is most easily distinguished from others, both biologically and clinically. CTF virus is a **reovirus** transmitted by the wood **tick** *Dermacentor andersoni* among the small **rodents**, e.g. chipmunks and squirrels, of the Rocky Mountains.
- West Nile virus (WNV) is a flavivirus that is classified in the same antigenic group as SLE virus. It is endemic in Africa but has caused encephalitis in areas of Europe and Asia as well. Wild birds are the main reservoir of this virus, which is transmitted by mosquitoes, especially *Culex* species. Humans are dead-end hosts. Transmission of the virus via solid organ transplants has also occurred.
- The clinical picture includes fever, contusion, and striking muscle weakness similar to that of Guillain-Barré syndrome in previously healthy people over the age of 60 years. Less than 1% of those infected have symptomatic disease.
- Prevention of yellow fever involves mosquito control and immunization with the **vaccine** containing live, attenuated yellow fever virus.
- Classic dengue (**breakbone fever**) begins suddenly with influenza-like syndrome consisting of fever, malaise, cough, and headache. Severe pains in muscles and joints (breakbone) occur. Enlarged lymph nodes, a maculopapular rash, and leukopenia are common. After a week or so, the symptoms regress but weakness may persist. Although unpleasant, this typical form of dengue is rarely fatal and has few sequelae.

  CMV Retinitis:
- Follicular center cell lymphoma
- *Cidofovir: no need of* PO_4
- *Fomivirsen:* first antisense antiviral approved by the FDA
- It is an oligonucleotide
- Intravitreal
- *Foscarnet*: inhibits viral DNA polymerases and reverse transcriptase

  No need of PO_4

↓ ↓ ↓

Calcium Potassium Magnesium

- *Trifluridine*: irreversible inhibitor of thymidylate synthase
- **Varicella**
- Fluorescent Antibody to Membrane Antigen (***FAMA***) – variable
- Varicella-Zoster IgG – within 4 days
- Prophylactic – 7 days after
- Incubation period – 10 to 21 days
- **EBV: Epstein-Barr virus**
- **Immunity reduced: CD4/CD8**
- EBV receptor: **complement C3d receptor** and **CD21** (cluster of differentiation 21) binds to antigens through attached C3d
- Cellular immunity is more important
- Hemolytic anemia
- Assoc. with 'Duncan's disease' or 'Purtilo syndrome' → **X-linked lymphoproliferative disease** (yet link between EBV not known)
- Sore throat, lymph node enlargement, rash
- Mixed cellularity
- **Lymphocyte-rich or lymphocytic predominance, Hodgkin's lymphoma**
- **Molluscum with antiretroviral treatment**

- **Topical Cidofovir**
- **Smallpox vaccination confers cross-protection**
- **Measles vaccine confers protection within 72 hours**
- **Parvovirus – B19 → IVIg**
- **HIV**
- 'c'– in India

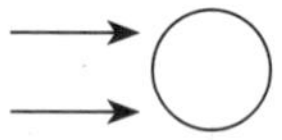

- Gp 120
- Gp 41
- **P^7 – Nuclei acid-binding protein**
- **P^{10} – Protease**
- **P^{24} – Capsid**
- **Tropical spastic paraparesis (TSP)**, also known as **HTLV-associated myelopathy (HAM)** or **chronic progressive myelopathy**
- ***HIV-associated nephropathy*** (HIVAN) – has Proteinuria
- Angiotensin-converting enzyme ***(ACE) inhibitiors are beneficial***
- ***Immune reconstitution in HIV with TB and $CD_4 < 50/\mu l$***
- Type 4 hypersensitivity
- Lymphadenopathy
- Fever
- Pulmonary infilteration — Treatment: ***Rx***

  ↑
- Increased intracranial tension (ICT) — Steriods
- Uveitis
- Graves' disease
- *Subcortical Dementia*
- 1st seizure: HIV encephalopathy
- MC seizure: ***Toxoplasmosis***

Kaposi:

- ***Intralesional vinblastin***
- ***PEG*** *Polyethylene glycol-coated*: **liposomal *doxorubicin (esp. in sec. Kaposi)***
- *(ABV)* → ***adriamycin, bleomycin, vincristine***

Antiretroviral Therapy (**ART**):

- Acute inflammatory syndrome
- Chronic symptomatic (nephropathy)
- Asymptomatic: $CD_4 < 350/\mu l$ and in pregnancy
- *Postexposure prophylaxis (PEP)*
- **PCP (**Pneumocystis pneumonia**)** *Prophylaxis:*
- $CD_4 < 200/\mu l$
- h/o PCP recovery
- Candidiasis
- **PEP – Candida + B**
- *Zidovudine + lamivudine + indinavir*: 4 weeks
- **HIV**
- MC helminthic – Strongyloides
- MC CNS infection – Cryptococcus
- HIV RNA and B_2 micro – Disease progress not CD_4
- Virion – Virus extracellular

- Virusoid – Nucleic acid dependent helper virus
- Viroid – Naked dsRNA
- Pseudovirion – Host capsid used for package

EBOLA

- *Biosafety – 4*
- *Negatively stained*
- *Filamentous virion*
- *Folded end-end: 'Bowl of Spaghetti'*
- *Liver necrosis – Councilman bodies*
- *Fever, Necrosis, Rash, Recrudescence.*

Robovirus

- *Hanta – Heart, Rodent*
- *HGE*: Human Granulocytic *Ehrlichia* – renal

Lassa Virus *(Rodents)*

- *Fetal death – 92%*
- *Male predominance*
- *Pericarditis*
- *Deafness*
- *Treatment: IV Ribavirin*

Dengue

- *Malnutrition protective*
- *Type 2 – more dangerous*
- *Female > Male*

Rabies

- *Incubation period: 1–3 months*
- *Encephalitis – 80%*
- *Paralytic – 20% (Ascending paralysis)*
- *Rabies immune globulin (RIG) within 7 days*
- *Postexposure: Intradermal PVRV rabies vaccine schedule*

@(days)	0	3	7	14	28	90
dose	2	2	2	0	1	1

- *Preexposure: rabies vaccine schedule*
- *@(days) 0, 7, 21/28.*
- *If previously vaccined: rabies vaccine schedule*
- *@(days) 0, 3.*
- *CAT II* *CAT II*

  Licks on Broken skin *Blood, Bat, Mucous.*
- *Remember: IPV (Injectable Polio Vaccine) - @(months) 0, 1, 6.*
- ***Atypical measles:*** A *formalin*-inactivated measles vaccine (**FIMV**) predisposed recipients to *atypical measles,* an immune complex-mediated disease.
- ***von Magnus phenomenon:*** The emergence of increasing quantities of low/noninfectious hemagglutinins seen in **influenza virus** (due to def. assembly)
- HSV – Brain Biopsy – Gold standard

- *Antigenic drift – Point mutation – immune selection*
- *Antigenic shift – Drastic change – major epidemic (10–15 years) → Influenza A only*
- **Hecht's pneumonia:** Also known as **giant cell pneumonia**, rare complication of **measles**
- ***Herpes***: *Syncytium (HSV-1)*
  Giant cells

Hepatitis:

- *Epidemiology: anti-HBC*
- *Hep [B] – 10^{-5} ml*
- *HCV: MC mode for Liver transplantation*
- *HCV RNA: Gold standard, no vaccine*
- *Hep E: Epidemic, pregnancy (10% mortality)*
  Precore mutants: *HbSAg +ve*
  HbeAg –ve
  Anti-HbeAg +ve
  Escape mutants: *HbeAg +ve*
  HbsAg –ve
- *HIV PCR gp 120*
- *gp 41* *any '2'*
- *gp 204*
- *gp 60*
- *No pol. needed*
- *Rabies and Rota virus } → Immunofluorescence*
- ***Eclipse period:*** *The time-interval between viral penetration and the production of progeny virions. (1st Progeny)*
- ***RSV*** – *No neuraminidase* and hemagglutinin – causes respiratory infection
- **Measles** – No *neuraminidase*

Mumps

- *Presternal Pitting edema*
- *Orchitis – 20% (15% – Bilateral)*
- *Sterility rare*
- *PORK-HAM – quantity*
- *HSV*
- *Variola*
- *Vaccinia* no chicken pox
- Cowpox
- Monkeypox
- *Plague – infectivity*

Pandas

- Pediatric autoimmune neuropsychiatric disorders associated with streptococcal infections
- *With OCD, Chorea, Tic*
- *Treatment: Penicillin/Azithromycin*

SSPE

- Subacute sclerosing pan encephalitis (*SSPE*) also known as Dawson disease, Dawson encephalitis, and measles encephalitis

- *Cowdry* type-A inclusion bodies
- *Myoclonic jerk*
- Synonyms for peptidoglycan are murein and mucopeptide.
- The carbohydrate backbone in a peptidoglycan is composed of alternating *N*-acetylmuramic acid and *N*-acetylglucosamine molecules. Attached to each of the muramic acid molecules is a tetrapeptide consisting of both D- and L-amino acids, the precise composition of which differs from one bacterium to another. Two of these amino acids are worthy of special mention: diaminopimelic acid, which is unique to bacterial cell walls, and D-alanine, which is involved in the cross-links between the tetrapeptides and in the action of penicillin. Note that this tetrapeptide contains the rare D-isomers of amino acids; most proteins contain the L-isomer. The other important component in this network is the peptide cross-link between the two tetrapeptides.
- *Teichoic acid*: These fibers of glycerol phosphate or ribitol phosphate are located in the outer layer of the gram-positive cell wall and extend from it. Some polymers of glycerol teichoic acid penetrate the peptidoglycan layer and are covalently linked to the lipid in the cytoplasmic membrane, in which case they are called lipoteichoic acid; others anchor to the muramic acid of the peptidoglycan.
- The most important naturally occurring compound is benzylpenicillin (penicillin G), which is composed of the 6-aminopenicillanic acid nucleus that all penicillins have, plus a benzyl side chain.
- Most cephalosporins are the products of molds of the genus *Cephalosporium;* a few, such as cefoxitin, are made by the actinomycete *Streptomyces.*
- Imipenem has the widest spectrum of activity of the β-lactam drugs. It has excellent bactericidal activity against many gram-positive, gram-negative, and anerobic bacteria. It is effective against most gram-positive cocci, e.g. streptococci and staphylococci; most gram-negative cocci, e.g. *Neisseria;* many gram-negative rods, e.g. *Pseudomonas, Haemophilus,* and members of the family Enterobacteriaceae, such as *E. coli;* and various, anerobes, e.g. *Bacteroides* and *Clostridium.* It is prescribed in combination with cilastatin, which is an inhibitor of dehydropeptidase, a kidney enzyme that inactivates imipenem. Imipenem is not inactivated by most β-lactamases.
- Two other carbapenems, ertapenem and meropenem, along with faropenem are available.
- Aztreonam, currently the most useful monobactam, has excellent activity against many gram-negative rods, such as *Enterobacteriaceae* and *Pseudomonas,* but is inactive against gram-positive and anerobic bacteria. It is resistant to most β-lactamases. It is very useful in patients who are hypersensitive to penicillin, because there is no cross-reactivity.
- Vancomycin is a glycopeptide that **inhibits cell wall synthesis by blocking transpeptidation** but by a mechanism different from that of the β-lactam drugs. Vancomycin binds directly to the D-alanyl-D-alanine portion of the pentapeptide which blocks the transpeptidase from binding, whereas the β-lactam drugs bind to the transpeptidase itself. Vancomycin also inhibits a second enzyme, the bacterial transglycosylase, which also functions in synthesizing the peptidoglycan, but this appears to be less important than inhibition of the transpeptidase.
- Apart from Staph. aureus, Vancomycin is also used in the treatment of infections caused by *Staphylococcus epidermidis* and enterococci. Strains of *S. aureus, S. epidermidis,* and enterococci with partial or complete resistance to vancomycin have been recovered from patients.
- Bacitracin is a cyclic polypeptide antibiotic that prevents the dephosphorylation of the phospholipid that carries the peptidoglycan subunit across the cell membrane. This blocks the regeneration of the lipid carrier and inhibits cell wall synthesis. Bacitracin is a bactericidal drug useful in the treatment of superficial skin infections but too toxic for systemic use.
- Chloramphenicol, clindamycin, linezolid and erythromycin act on the 50S subunit. Remember CCLEaner.
- *Calymmatobacterium granulomatis* is a gram-negative rod that causes granuloma inguinale, a sexually transmitted disease characterized by genital ulceration and soft tissue and bone destruction. The diagnosis is made by visualizing the stained organisms (Donovan bodies) within large macrophages from the lesion. Tetracycline is the treatment of choice for this disease, which is rare in the United States but endemic in many developing countries.

- Tetracyclines are a family of antibiotics with bacteriostatic activity against a variety of gram-positive and gram-negative bacteria, mycoplasmas, chlamydiae, and rickettsiae.
- Chloramphenicol is active against a broad range of organisms, including gram-positive and gram-negative bacteria (including anerobes). It is bacteriostatic against certain organisms, such as *Salmonella typhi,* but has bactericidal activity against the three important encapsulated organisms that cause meningitis: *Haemophilus influenzae, Streptococcus pneumoniae,* and *Neisseria meningitidis.*
- Aminoglycosides are bactericidal drugs especially useful against many gram-negative rods. Certain aminoglycosides are used against other organisms; e.g. streptomycin is used in the multidrug therapy of tuberculosis, tularemia, plague, brucellosis, and gentamicin is used in combination with penicillin G against enterococci.
- Erythromycin is a bacteriostatic drug with a wide spectrum of activity. It is the treatment of choice for pneumonia caused by *Legionella* (a gram-negative rod) and *Mycoplasma* (a wall-less bacterium) and is also an effective alternative against a variety of infections caused by gram-positive cocci in penicillin-allergic patients.
- *Clindamycin*: The most useful clinical activity of this bacteriostatic drug is against anerobes, both gram-positive bacteria, such as *Clostridium perfringens* and gram-negative bacteria, such as *Bacteroides fragilis.* The most important side effect of clindamycin is pseudomembranous colitis.
- Linezolid is useful for the treatment of vancomycin-resistant enterococci, methicillin-resistant *S. aureus* and *S. epidermidis,* and penicillin-resistant pneumococci. It is bacteriostatic against enterococci and staphylococci but bactericidal against pneumococci.
- Telithromycin (Ketek) is the first clinically useful member of the ketolide group of antibiotics. It is similar to the macrolides in general structure and mode of action but is sufficiently different chemically, that organisms resistant to macrolides may be sensitive to telithromycin. It has a wide spectrum of activity against a variety of gram-positive and gram-negative bacteria (including macrolide-resistant pneumococci) and is used in the treatment of community-acquired pneumonia, bronchitis, and sinusitis.
- A combination of two streptogramins, quinopristin and dalfopristin (Synercid), is used for the treatment of bloodstream infections caused by vancomycin-resistant *Enterococcus faecium* (but not vancomycin-resistant *Enterococcus faecalis*). It is also approved for use in skin infections caused by *Streptococcus pyogenes* and by methicillin-sensitive *Staphylococcus aureus.*
- Either alone or in combination with trimethoprim, sulfonamides are useful in a variety of bacterial diseases, such as urinary tract infections caused by *Escherichia coli,* otitis media caused by *S. pneumoniae* or *H. influenzae* in children, shigellosis, nocardiosis, and chancroid. In combination, they are also the drugs of choice for two protozoan diseases, toxoplasmosis and *Pneumocystis* pneumonia.
- Trimethoprim-sulfamethoxazole is clinically useful in the treatment of urinary tract infections, *Pneumocystis* pneumonia, and shigellosis. It also is used for prophylaxis in granulopenic patients to prevent opportunistic infections.
- Fluoroquinolones are active against a broad range of organisms that cause infections of the lower respiratory tract, intestinal tract, urinary tract, and skeletal and soft tissues. Fluoroquinolones should not be given to pregnant women and young children because they damage growing bone.
- In the United States, there are two rickettsial diseases of significance: Rocky Mountain spotted fever, caused by *Rickettsia rickettsii,* and Q fever, caused by *Coxiella burnetii.* Several other rickettsial diseases, such as epidemic, endemic, and scrub typhus are important in the developing countries. Rickettsialpox, caused by *Rickettsia akari,* is a rare disease found in certain densely populated cities in the United States.
- The treatment of choice for all rickettsial diseases is tetracycline, with chloramphenicol as the second choice.
- *C. trachomatis* exists in more than 15 immunotypes (A–L). Types A, B, and C cause **trachoma**, a chronic conjunctivitis endemic in Africa and Asia. Types D–K cause **genital tract infections,** which are occasionally transmitted to the eyes or the respiratory tract. *C. trachomatis* L1–L3 immunotypes cause **lymphogranuloma venereum,** a sexually transmitted disease with lesions on genitalia and in lymph nodes.
- All chlamydiae are susceptible to tetracyclines, such as doxycycline, and macrolides, such as erythromycin and azithromycin. The drug of choice for *C. trachomatis* sexually transmitted diseases is azithromycin. Because the rate of coinfection with gonococci and *C. trachomatis* is high, any patient with a diagnosis of gonorrhea should also be treated for *C. trachomatis* with azithromycin. The drug of choice for neonatal inclusion conjunctivitis

is erythromycin. The drug of choice for *C. psittaci* and *C. pneumoniae* infections and for lymphogranuloma venereum is a tetracycline, such as doxycycline.

- *M. pneumoniae* causes 'atypical' pneumonia. The colony frequently has a characteristic 'fried-egg' shape, with a raised center and a thinner outer edge. *Mycoplasma* pneumonia is the most common type of atypical pneumonia. It was formerly called **primary atypical pneumonia.** (Other atypical pneumonias are Legionnaires 'disease, Q fever, psittacosis, and viral pneumonias such as influenza. The term 'atypical' means that a causative bacterium cannot be isolated on routine media in the diagnostic laboratory or that the disease does not resemble pneumococcal pneumonia.)
- The treatment of choice is either a macrolide, such as erythromycin or azithromycin, or a tetracycline, such as doxycycline. These drugs can shorten the duration of symptoms, although, as mentioned above, the disease resolves spontaneously. Penicillins and cephalosporins are **inactive** because the organism has no cell wall.
- *Mycoplasma hominis* has been implicated as an infrequent cause of pelvic inflammatory disease. *Ureaplasma urealyticum* may cause approximately 20% of cases of nongonococcal urethritis. Ureaplasmas can be distinguished from mycoplasmas by their ability to produce the enzyme urease, which degrades urea to ammonia and carbon dioxide.
- Actinomycetes are true bacteria (related to corynebacteria and mycobacteria), but they form **long, branching filaments** that resemble the hyphae of fungi. They are gram-positive, but some (such as *Nocardia asteroides*) are also weakly acid-fast. Actinomyces are anerobic; treatment consists of prolonged administration of penicillin G, coupled with surgical drainage. There is no significant resistance to penicillin G. Nocardia are aerobic. Treatment is with trimethoprim-sulfamethoxazole. Surgical drainage may also be needed. Occasional drug resistance occurs. No vaccine or prophylactic drug is available.
- *T. pallidum* grows **very slowly**. The medical importance of that fact is that antibiotics must be present at an effective level for several weeks to kill the organisms and cure the disease. For example, benzathine penicillin is the form of penicillin used to treat primary and secondary syphilis because the penicillin is released very slowly from this depot preparation and bactericidal concentrations are present for weeks after administration of the antibiotic. If the patient is allergic to penicillin, doxycycline can be used but must be given for prolonged periods to effect a cure. In neurosyphilis, high doses of aqueous penicillin G are administered because benzathine penicillin penetrates poorly into the central nervous system.
- The nonvenereal treponemal diseases include bejel in Africa, yaws (caused by *T. pallidum* subspecies *pertenue*) in many humid tropical countries and pinta (caused by *Treponema carateum*) in Central and South America. All can be cured by penicillin.
- *B. burgdorferi* is transmitted by tick bite. The tick *Ixodes scapularis* is the vector. The major bacterial diseases transmitted by ticks in the United States are Lyme disease, Rocky Mountain spotted fever, ehrlichiosis, relapsing fever, and tularemia. *I. scapularis* ticks transmit three diseases: two bacterial diseases, Lyme disease and human granulocytic ehrlichiosis, and the protozoan disease, babesiosis. The treatment of choice for stage 1 disease or other mild manifestations is either doxycycline or amoxicillin. For more severe forms or late-stage disease, ceftriaxone is recommended. There is no significant antibiotic resistance.
- *B. recurrentis* is transmitted from person to person by the **human body louse**. Humans are the only hosts. *B. hermsii* and many other *Borrelia* species are transmitted to humans by soft **ticks** (*Ornithodoros*). Tetracycline may be beneficial early in the illness and may prevent relapses.
- *Leptospira interrogans* is the cause of leptospirosis. The treatment of choice is penicillin G. Doxycycline is effective in preventing the disease in exposed persons.
- *Spirillum minor* causes one type of rat bite fever in humans. *Streptobacillus moniliformis,* a gram-negative rod, also causes rat bite fever.
- *Bartonella* species are pleomorphic gram-negative rods. *Bartonella henselae* (formerly called *Rochalimaea henselae*) is the cause of **Bacillary angiomatosis** and **Cat-scratch fever**. It is characterized by proliferative, vascular lesions resembling Kaposi's sarcoma in the skin and visceral organs. The organism can be visualized in the biopsy tissue using the Warthin-Starry silver stain. Treatment with doxycycline or erythromycin is effective. (Bacillary peliosis is similar to bacillary angiomatosis except that in peliosis, the lesions occur primarily in the liver and spleen.)

- *Bartonella quintana* (formerly called *Rochalimaea quintana*) is the cause of trench fever and also is implicated as the cause of some cases of bacillary angiomatosis.
- *Ehrlichia chaffeensis* is a member of the rickettsia family and causes human monocytic ehrlichiosis (HME). This disease resembles Rocky Mountain spotted fever, except that the typical rash usually does not occur. *E. chaffeensis* primarily infects mononuclear leukocytes and forms characteristic **morulae** in the cytoplasm. (A morula is an inclusion body that resembles a mulberry. It consists of many *E. chaffeensis* cells.) Doxycycline is the treatment of choice.
- The name 'HACEK' is an acronym of the first letters of the genera of the following bacteria: *Haemophilus aphrophilus* and *Haemophilus paraphrophilus, Actinobacillus actinomycetemcomitans, Cardiobacterium hominis, Eikenella corrodens,* and *Kingella kingae.*
- Haemophilus ducreyi causes the sexually transmitted disease **chancroid** (soft chancre). Chancroid can be treated with erythromycin, azithromycin, or ceftriaxone.
- *Moraxella* species are gram-negative coccobacillary rods resembling neisseriae. *M. catarrhalis* is the major pathogen in this genus. It causes otitis media and sinusitis, primarily in children, as well as bronchitis and pneumonia in older people with chronic obstructive pulmonary disease. Trimethoprim-sulfamethoxazole or amoxicillin-clavulanate can be used to treat these infections. *Moraxella nonliquefaciens* is one of the two common causes of blepharitis (infection of the eyelid); *Staphylococcus aureus* is the other. The usual treatment is local application of antibiotic ointment, such as erythromycin.
- *Brucella* species cause brucellosis (undulant fever). Brucellae are small gram-negative rods without a capsule. The three major human pathogens and their animal reservoirs are *Brucella melitensis* (goats and sheep), *Brucella abortus* (cattle), and *Brucella suis* (pigs). The undulating (rising-and-falling) fever pattern that gives the disease its name occurs in a minority of patients. Enlarged lymph nodes, liver, and spleen are frequently found. Pancytopenia occurs. *B. melitensis* infections tend to be more severe and prolonged, whereas those caused by *B. abortus* are more self-limited. Osteomyelitis is the most frequent complication. The treatment of choice is tetracycline plus rifampin. There is no significant resistance to these drugs.
- *F. tularensis* is a small, pleomorphic gram-negative rod. Approximately 75% of cases are the 'ulceroglandular' type, in which the site of entry ulcerates and the regional lymph nodes are swollen and painful. Other, less frequent forms of tularemia include glandular, oculoglandular, typhoidal, gastrointestinal, and pulmonary. Disease usually confers lifelong immunity. Attempts to culture the organism in the laboratory are rarely undertaken, because there is a high risk to laboratory workers of infection by inhalation and the special cysteine-containing medium required for growth is not usually available. Streptomycin is the drug of choice. There is no significant antibiotic resistance.
- *Y. pestis* is a small gram-negative rod that exhibits bipolar staining. Untreated bubonic plague is fatal in approximately half of the cases, and untreated pneumonic plague is invariably fatal. The treatment of choice is a combination of streptomycin and tetracycline, although streptomycin alone can be used. There is no significant antibiotic resistance. In view of the rapid progression of the disease, treatment should not wait for the results of the bacteriologic culture. Incision and drainage of the buboes are not usually necessary.
- *Pasteurella multocida* causes wound infections (rapidly spreading cellulitis) associated with cat and dog bites. *P. multocida* is a short, encapsulated gram-negative rod that exhibits bipolar staining. Osteomyelitis can complicate cat bites in particular, because cats' sharp, pointed teeth can implant the organism under the periosteum. Penicillin G is the treatment of choice. There is no significant antibiotic resistance.
- The endotoxin of *N. meningitidis* is a lipo**poly**saccharide (LPS) similar to that found in many gram-negative rods, but the endotoxin of *N. gonorrhoeae* is a lipo**oligo**saccharide (LOS). For meningitis, use penicillin G. In uncomplicated gonococcal infections, ceftriaxone is the treatment of choice. Spectinomycin or ciprofloxacin should be used if the patient is allergic to penicillin. Because mixed infections with *C. trachomatis* are common, tetracycline should also be prescribed.
- *H. influenzae* used to be the leading cause of meningitis in young children, but the use of the highly effective 'conjugate' vaccine has greatly reduced the incidence of meningitis caused by this organism.
- Growth of the organism on laboratory media requires the addition of two components, **heme (factor X)** and **NAD (factor V),** for adequate energy production. Rarely, **epiglottitis,** which can obstruct the airway, occurs.

This life-threatening disease of young children is caused almost exclusively by *H. influenzae.* The treatment of choice for meningitis or other serious systemic infections caused by H. influenzae is ceftriaxone.

- *H. influenzae* upper respiratory tract infections, such as otitis media and sinusitis, are treated with either amoxicillin-clavulanate or trimethoprim-sulfamethoxazole. Meningitis in close contacts of the patient can be prevented by rifampin. Rifampin is used because it is secreted in the saliva to a greater extent than ampicillin. Rifampin decreases respiratory carriage of the organism, thereby reducing transmission.
- *B. pertussis* is a small, coccobacillary, encapsulated gram-negative rod is pathogen **only for humans**, is transmitted by **airborne droplets** produced during the severe coughing episodes. The organisms attach to the ciliated epithelium of the upper respiratory tract but do not invade the underlying tissue. Erythromycin reduces the number of organisms in the throat and decreases the risk of secondary complications but has little influence on the course of the disease because the toxins have already damaged the respiratory mucosa.
- *L. pneumophila* (and other legionellae) causes pneumonia, both in the community and in hospitalized immunocompromised patients. Legionellae are gram-negative rods that **stain faintly with the standard Gram stain**. Legionellae in lung biopsy sections do not stain by the standard hematoxylin-and-eosin (HandE) procedure; therefore, special methods, such as the Dieterle silver impregnation stain, are used to visualize the organisms.
- Legionellae are associated chiefly with **environmental water sources**. The typical candidate for Legionnaire's disease is an older man who smokes and consumes substantial amounts of alcohol. The clinical picture can vary from a mild influenza-like illness to a severe pneumonia accompanied by mental confusion, nonbloody diarrhea, proteinuria, and microscopic hematuria. Pontiac fever is a mild, flu-like form of *Legionella* infection that does not result in pneumonia. Charcoal-yeast agar, a special medium supplemented with iron and cysteine is used for culture. The cold-agglutinin titer does not rise in *Legionella* pneumonia, in contrast to pneumonia caused by *Mycoplasma.*
- Azithromycin or erythromycin (with or without rifampin) is the treatment of choice. Certain fluoroquinolones, such as levofloxacin and trovafloxacin, are also drugs of choice. These drugs are effective not only against L. pneumophila but also against Mycoplasma pneumoniae and Streptococcus pneumoniae. The organism frequently produces β-lactamase, and so penicillins and cephalosporins are less effective.
- *B. anthracis* is a large gram-positive rod with square ends, frequently found in chains. After being inhaled into the lung, the organism moves rapidly to the mediastinal lymph nodes, where it causes hemorrhagic mediastinitis. Ciprofloxacin is the drug of choice. Doxycycline is an alternative drug.
- *C. perfringens* causes two distinct diseases, gas gangrene and food poisoning, depending on the route of entry into the body. Penicillin G is the antibiotic of choice.
- Diphtheria toxin inhibits protein synthesis by **ADP-ribosylation of elongation factor 2** (EF-2). The DNA that codes for diphtheria toxin is part of the genetic material of a temperate bacteriophage. The immune status of a person can be assessed by Schick's test. The test is performed by intradermal injection of 0.1 mL of purified standardized toxin. If the patient has no antitoxin, the toxin will cause inflammation at the site 4–7 days later. A throat swab should be cultured on Löffler's medium, a **tellurite plate,** and a blood agar plate. The treatment of choice is **antitoxin**. Treatment with penicillin G or an erythromycin is recommended also.
- *L. monocytogenes* causes meningitis and sepsis in newborns, pregnant women, and immunosuppressed adults. It also causes outbreaks of febrile gastroenteritis. *Listeria* grows well at cold temperatures, so storage of contaminated food in the refrigerator can increase the risk of gastroenteritis. This paradoxical growth in the cold is called 'cold enhancement'. Treatment of invasive disease, such as meningitis and sepsis, consists of trimethoprim-sulfamethoxazole. Combinations, such as ampicillin and gentamicin or ampicillin and trimethoprim-sulfamethoxazole, can also be used. Resistant strains are rare.
- The treatment of choice for enteric fevers, such as typhoid fever and septicemia with metastatic infection is either ceftriaxone or ciprofloxacin. Ampicillin or ciprofloxacin should be used in patients who are chronic carriers of *S. typhi.*
- The main treatment for shigellosis is fluid and electrolyte replacement. In mild cases, no antibiotics are indicated. In severe cases, a fluoroquinolone (e.g. ciprofloxacin) is the drug of choice, but the incidence of plasmids conveying multiple drug resistance is high enough that antibiotic sensitivity tests must be performed. Trimethoprim-sulfamethoxazole is an alternative choice.

- Erythromycin or ciprofloxacin is used successfully in *C. jejuni* enterocolitis. The treatment of choice for *C. intestinalis* bacteremia is an aminoglycoside.
- *Klebsiella-Enterobacter-Serratia* Group: These organisms are usually opportunistic pathogens that cause nosocomial infections, especially pneumonia and urinary tract infections. *Klebsiella pneumoniae* is an important respiratory tract pathogen outside hospitals as well. *Klebsiella* produces thick, bloody sputum ('currant-jelly' sputum) and can progress to necrosis and abscess formation. *K. Pneumoniae, enterobacter cloacae,* and *serratia marcescens* are the species most often involved in human infections. An aminoglycoside, e.g. gentamicin, and a cephalosporin, e.g. cefotaxime, are used empirically until the results of testing are known.
- *Proteus-providencia-morganella* group: These organisms primarily cause urinary tract infections, both community- and hospital-acquired. *Proteus* species can also cause pneumonia, wound infections, and septicemia. Most strains are sensitive to aminoglycosides and trimethoprim-sulfamethoxazole.
- *Pseudomonas aeruginosa* causes infections (e.g. sepsis, pneumonia, and urinary tract infections) primarily in patients with lowered host defenses. Pathogenesis is based on multiple virulence factors: endotoxin, exotoxins, and enzymes. Its endotoxin, like that of other gram-negative bacteria, causes the symptoms of sepsis and septic shock. The best known of the exotoxins is exotoxin A, which causes tissue necrosis. It inhibits eukaryotic protein synthesis by the same mechanism as diphtheria exotoxin, namely ADP-ribosylation of elongation factor 2. Pyocyanin damages the cilia and mucosal cells of the respiratory tract. Exo S has several modes of action, the most important of which is ADP-ribosylation of a Ras protein, leading to damage to the cytoskeleton. The bacteria can spread to the skin, where they cause black, necrotic lesions called **ecthyma gangrenosum**. Severe external otitis **(malignant otitis externa)** and other skin lesions (e.g. **folliculitis**) occur in users of swimming pools and hot tubs in which the chlorination is inadequate. *P. aeruginosa* is the most common cause of **osteochondritis** of the foot in those who sustain puncture wounds through the soles of gym shoes. **Corneal infections** caused by *P. aeruginosa* are seen in contact lens users. Because *P. aeruginosa* is **resistant to many antibiotics**, treatment must be tailored to the sensitivity of each isolate and monitored frequently; resistant strains can emerge during therapy. The treatment of choice is an antipseudomonal penicillin, e.g. ticarcillin or piperacillin, plus an aminoglycoside, e.g. gentamicin or amikacin.
- *B. fragilis* members are resistant to penicillins, first-generation cephalosporins, and aminoglycosides, making them among the most antibiotic-resistant of the anerobic bacteria. Penicillin resistance is the result of β-lactamase production. Metronidazole is the drug of choice, with cefoxitin, clindamycin, and chloramphenicol as alternatives.

CHAPTER 7

Pathology

MAJOR HISTOCOMPATIBILITY COMPLEX (MHC)/HUMAN LEUKOCYTE ANTIGEN (HLA)

Class I	Class II	Class III
• HLA-ABCEF • MHC-I-beta 2 microglobulin • All nucleated cells and platelets • CD8 T cells • Virus infected cels • Graft rejection • Cell mediated cytolysis	• HLA-D • B cells • Macrophages • APCs • CD 4 • GVHD • Mixed leucocyte reaction	• C2 C4 complement • TNF alpha and beta • HSP • Properdin • 21-hydroxylase

Acute Phase Reactants

- Alpha 1 antitrypsin
- CRP
- Fibrinogen
- Alpha one acid glycoprotein
- Haptoglobulin

Psammoma Bodies

- Papillary ca thyroid
- Meningioma
- Pituitary adenoma
- Serous cystadenoma
- RCC
- Appendiceal ca

SPHEROCYTOSIS AND RBC MEMBRANE

Ankyrin	MCC of hereditary spherocytosis
Spectrin	MCC of elliptocytosis
Protein 3	Anion transport channel
Protein 4.2	Palladin
Protein 4.1	Combines with glycophorin A

Pattern

- Palisade: Schwann cell
- Storiform: Fibrohistiocytic
- Herring bone: Fibrosarcoma
- Right angle: Smooth muscle
- Biphasic: Synovial sarcoma

Small Round Blue Cell Tumors

- Neuroblastoma
- Ewings sarcoma
- Non-Hodgkin's lymphoma
- Askin tumor (PNET)
- Wilms tumor
- Rhabdomyosarcoma
- Primitive neuroectodermal

Mallory Hyaline

- Alcoholic liver disease
- Indian childhood cirrhosis
- Wilson's disease
- Focal nodular hyperplasia
- Primary biliary cirrhosis
- Alpha one antitrypsin deficiency
- Hepatocellular Ca

Small Cell Ca

- GRP
- AVP (ADH)
- Calcitonin
- ACTH
- ANF

Paraneoplastic Syndromes

Hypoglycemia

- Fibrosarcoma
- HCC

Hyperglycemia

- Osteosarcoma

Hypercalcemia

- Squamous cell ca of lung
- Renal Ca
- Adult T cell
- Breast Ca
- Ovarian Ca

Myasthenia

- Bronchogenic Ca

Acanthosis nigricans

- Gastric Ca
- Breast Ca
- Lung Ca
- Uterine Ca

AL (amyloid light chain)
- Primary amyloidosis
- Multiple myeloma

AA (Amyloid associated protein)
- Chronic infection and inflammation
- Ca-renal cell carcinoma
- Connective tissue disorder
- Hodgkin's lymphoma

Abeta 2 microglobulin
- Hemodialysis

AB
- Beta 2 amyloid in senile cerebral, Alzheimer's

AIAPP-Type 2 DM

ATTR- Transthyretin
- Familial amyloidosis
- Neuropathy
- Systemic senile amyloidosis

ACAL-calcitonin
- Medullary Ca thyroid

AANF (Atrial Natriuretic Factor Associated)
- Isolated atrial amyloidosis
- Prion disease

TUMOR MARKERS

Tumor marker	Condition
HMB 45, S100, Ki55	Melanoma
HAM 56, CD 68, Factor 13 A, Lysozyme	Fibrohistiocytic tumor
Mel cam, Ki6, 7	Placental site trophoblastic tumor
CD 31, (PECAM), factor 8, CD 62, Selectin	Kaposis sarcoma, vascular tumors
CD 117, C kit, CD 34, SM actin	GIST
CD 57, NSE, Chromogranin, synaptophysin	Neuroblastoma, adrenal medulla tumors
Catretinin, epi membrane antigen (EMA)	Mesothelioma
D actin, desmin, myo D1	Rhabdomyosarcoma
Carbonic anhydrase C	Oligodendrocyte
Osteocalcin > osteonectin	Osteosarcoma
Osteopontin	Brain, kidney, ovarian epithelial tumors
E cadherin	Lost in lobular invasive Ca
CD 55- decay accelerating factor CD 58 CD 59- membrane inhibition of reactive lysis	PNH
CD 43, CD117, MPO	Chloroma
CD 13, CD 33, CD 117, MPO	Monocyte macro (myeloid)
CD 1a, S100, HLA DR, Langerin, CD 207	Langhans histocytosis
CD 2	Measle
CD 3	Pan T cell, NK cell
CD 8/11 ICAM	Neutrophil
CD 21	EBV receptor
CD 56, 16	NK cell
CD 41, 61	Platelet
CD 13, 33115, 116, 117	Myeloid
CD 15, 30	Hodgkin's
P 73	Extranodal NK/T cell
P53	Endometrial ca, anaplastic Ca
P57	Absent in complete mole
GLUT 1	Epithelia ovarian tumors

Ca 15 3	Breast Ca
Ca 19 9	Pancreas colon breat
CD 34	Pluropotent
CD 43	Marginal zone, chloroma
CD 45	LCA
CD 10	CALLA
CD 62	Selectin
CD 95	Apoptein
Annexin V	Thrombospondin
CD 103	Hairy cell leukemia
CD 99	Ewing's sarcoma
MET	Follicular Ca thyroid
RET	Medullary Ca thyroid
TRK	Papillary Ca thyroid
S100	Sustenticular cell, melanoma
Vit.B12 binding globulin, neurotensin, AFP	Melanoma
Vimentin	Seminoma Sarcoma Melanoma Lymphoma
CEA	Colon Pancreas Lung Stomach Heart
CA 125	Epi Ca ovary Adenocarcinoma cervix Endometrial Ca GIT tumor
Keratin	Carcinoma Mesothelioma

Chromosome

No.	Disease
1	P73, neuroblastoma
3	VHL
4	Huntingtons, ADPKD
6	ARPKD
7	Cystic fibrosis
9	Tuberous sclerosis
11	Ataxia telangiectsia
13	Wilsons, BRCA1, RB
17	P53, NF1, BRCA2
21	Folate transporter
22	NF2

Microdeletion

11 p 13	WAGR
13 q 14.1	RB
15 q 18.13	Prader willi, Angelman
17 p 13.13	Miller dieker/Criduchat
22 q 11	DiGeorge/velocardiofacial syndrome

CKD with normal sized kidneys

- Amyloidosis
- Multiple myeloma
- Diabetic nephropathy
- ADPKD
- RPGN
- Obstructive nephropathy

Cell Injury

Reversible cell injury	Irreversible cell injury
Blebbing of plasma membrane ↓ Swelling of endoplasmic reticulum and mitochondria ↓ Detachment of ribosomes ↓ Clumping of chromatin ***Loss of microvilli*** ***Myelin figures***	Increased swelling of plasma membrane Disruption of cellular membrane Swelling and disruption of lysosome Amorphous densities in mitochondria Pyknosis (Nuclear condensation) Karyorrhexis (Nulcear fragmentation) Karyolysis (Dissolution of nucleus)

Hematology

- Aplastic anemia age distribution is biphasic, with the major peak in the teens and twenties and a second rise in older adults.
- Radiation dosimetry is the measurement and calculation of the radiation dose received by matter and tissue resulting from the exposure to indirect and direct ionizing radiation.
- Benzene is a notorious cause of bone marrow failure.
- Drugs consistently producing aplastic anemia: *Benzene, Chloramphenicol, quinacrine and chloroquine, mepacrine, phenylbutazone, hydantoins, carbamazepine, gold, cimetidine, d-penicillamine.*
- Hepatitis is the most common preceding infection for aplastic anemia, and posthepatitis marrow failure accounts for approximately 5% of etiologies in most series. The hepatitis is seronegative (non-A, non-B, non-C) and possibly due to an as yet undiscovered infectious agent.
- Aplastic anemia is strongly associated with the rare collagen vascular syndrome *eosinophilic fasciitis* that is characterized by painful induration of subcutaneous tissues.
- Fanconi's anemia, an autosomal recessive disorder, manifests as congenital developmental anomalies, progressive pancytopenia, and an increased risk of malignancy.
- Chromosomes in Fanconi's anemia are peculiarly susceptible to DNA cross-linking agents, the basis for a diagnostic assay.

- Patients with Fanconi's anemia typically have short stature, café au lait spots, and anomalies involving the thumb, radius, and genitourinary tract. At least 12 different genetic defects (all but one with an identified gene) have been defined; the most common, type A Fanconi's anemia, is due to a mutation in *FANCA*.
- Dyskeratosis congenita is characterized by mucous membrane leukoplakia, dystrophic nails, reticular hyperpigmentation, and the development of aplastic anemia in childhood.
- Dyskeratosis is due to mutations in genes of the telomere repair complex, which acts to maintain telomere length in replicating cells: The X-linked variety is due to mutations in the *DKC1* (*dyskerin*) gene; the more unusual autosomal dominant type is due to mutation in *TERC*, which encodes an RNA template, and *TERT*, which encodes the catalytic reverse transcriptase, telomerase. Mutations in TNF2, a component of the shelterin, proteins that bind the telomere DNA, also occur in dyskeratosis.
- In Shwachman-Diamond syndrome, marrow failure is seen with pancreatic insufficiency and malabsorption; most patients have compound heterozygous mutations in *SBDS* that may affect marrow stroma function.
- Cells bearing the CD34 antigen, a marker of early hematopoietic cells, are greatly diminished.
- Infection is an unusual first symptom in aplastic anemia (unlike in agranulocytosis, where pharyngitis, anorectal infection, or frank sepsis occur early). A striking feature of aplastic anemia is the restriction of symptoms to the hematologic system, and patients often feel and look remarkably well despite drastically reduced blood counts.
- Lymphadenopathy and splenomegaly are highly atypical of aplastic anemia. Café au lait spots and short stature suggest Fanconi's anemia; peculiar nails and leukoplakia suggest dyskeratosis congenita.
- Chromosome breakage studies of peripheral blood using diepoxybutane or mitomycin C should be performed on children and younger adults to exclude Fanconi's anemia.
- Typhlitis is necrotizing colitis.
- Agranulocytosis has an incidence similar to aplastic anemia but is especially frequent among older adults and in women.
- Diamond-Blackfan anemia, or congenital PRCA (Pure Red Cell Aplasia), is diagnosed at birth or in early childhood and often responds to glucocorticoid treatment; mutations in ribosomal RNA processing genes are etiologic.
- PRCA has important associations with immune system diseases.
- *Parvovirus:* The bone marrow shows red cell aplasia and the presence of giant pronormoblasts, which is the cytopathic sign of B19 parvovirus infection. Viral tropism for human erythroid progenitor cells is due to its use of erythrocyte P antigen as a cellular receptor for entry.
- Secondary MDS occurs as a late toxicity of cancer treatment, usually with a combination of radiation and the radiomimetic alkylating agents such as busulfan, nitrosourea, or procarbazine (with a latent period of 5–7 years) or the DNA topoisomerase inhibitors (2 years)
- Cytogenetic abnormalities are not random (loss of all or part of 5, 7, and 20, trisomy of 8) and may be related to etiology (11q23 following topoisomerase II inhibitors); CMML is often associated with t(5;12) that creates a chimeric *tel-PDGF* β gene. Mutations of N-*ras* (an oncogene), *p53* and *IRF-1* (tumor suppressor genes), *Bcl-2* (an antiapoptotic gene), and others have been reported in some patients but likely occur late in the sequence leading to leukemic transformation. Sideroblastic anemia may be related to mutations in mitochondrial genes
- Children with Down syndrome are susceptible to MDS, and a family history may indicate a hereditary form of sideroblastic anemia or Fanconi's anemia.
- The physical examination is remarkable for signs of anemia; approximately 20% of patients have splenomegaly. Some unusual skin lesions, including Sweet's syndrome (febrile neutrophilic dermatosis), occur with MDS.
- The WHO considers the presence of 20% blasts in the marrow as the criterion that separates acute myeloid leukemia (AML) from MDS.
- Most patients die as a result of complications of pancytopenia and not due to leukemic transformation; perhaps one-third will succumb to other diseases unrelated to their MDS.
- Precipitous worsening of pancytopenia, acquisition of new chromosomal abnormalities on serial cytogenetic determination, increase in the number of blasts, and marrow fibrosis are all poor prognostic indicators.
- Azacitidine is directly cytotoxic but also inhibits DNA methylation, thereby altering gene expression.

- Decitabine is closely related to azacitidine and more potent.
- Lenalidomide, a thalidomide derivative with a more favorable toxicity profile, is particularly effective in reversing anemia in MDS patients with 5q—syndrome. Toxicities include myelosuppression (worsening thrombocytopenia and neutropenia, necessitating blood count monitoring) and an increased risk of deep vein thrombosis and pulmonary embolism.
- Fibrosis of the bone marrow usually accompanied by a characteristic blood smear picture called *leukoerythroblastosis*, can occur as a primary hematologic disease, called *myelofibrosis* or *myeloid metaplasia* and as a secondary process, called *myelophthisis*.
- CML is the consequence of the balanced translocation between chromosomes 9 and 22 [t(9;22)(q34;11)]
- CNL has been associated with a t(15;19) translocation.
- CEL occurs with a deletion or balanced translocations involving the *PDGFR* α gene.
- By contrast, to a greater or lesser extent, PV, PMF, and ET are characterized by expression of a *JAK2* mutation.
- Importantly, the *JAK2* gene is located on the short arm of chromosome 9, and loss of heterozygosity on chromosome 9p, due to mitotic recombination is the most common cytogenetic abnormality in PV.
- With the exception of aquagenic pruritus, no symptoms distinguish PV from other causes of erythrocytosis.
- Relative erythrocytosis due to a reduction in plasma volume alone is known as *stress* or *spurious erythrocytosis* or *Gaisböck's syndrome.*
- Only three situations cause microcytic erythrocytosis: β-thalassemia trait, hypoxic erythrocytosis, and PV.
- *Erythromelalgia* is a curious syndrome of unknown etiology associated with thrombocytosis, primarily involving the lower extremities and usually manifested by erythema, warmth, and pain of the affected appendage and occasionally digital infarction. It occurs with a variable frequency in MPD patients and is usually responsive to salicylates.
- Pegylated IFN-α produces complete remission in PV patients and its role in this disorder may be expanding.
- Anagrelide, a phosphodiesterase inhibitor, can reduce the platelet count and, if tolerated, is preferable to hydroxyurea because it lacks marrow toxicity and actually is protective against venous thrombosis.
- An intriguing feature of PMF is the occurrence of autoimmune abnormalities such as immune complexes, antinuclear antibodies, rheumatoid factor, or a positive Coombs' test.
- For unknown reasons, the number of circulating CD34+ cells is markedly increased in PMF (> 15, 000/µl) compared to the other chronic MPDs, unless they too develop myeloid metaplasia.
- Survival in PMF varies according to specific clinical features (Table 108–4) but is shorter than in patients with PV or ET.
- Important prognostic factors for disease acceleration include anemia, leukocytosis, thrombocytopenia, the presence of circulating myeloblasts, older age, the presence of complex cytogenetic abnormalities, and constitutional symptoms such as unexplained fever, night sweats, or weight loss.
- There is an unexplained female predominance in contrast to PMF or the reactive forms of thrombocytosis where no sex difference exists.
- Iron deficiency anemia can produce an increase in the number of platelets!! As does ethanol abuse!!
- Mpl is the receptor for thrombopoietin.
- As in the case of early erythroid and myeloid progenitor cells, early megakaryocytic progenitors require the presence of interleukin 3 (IL-3) and stem cell factor for optimal proliferation in addition to thrombopoietin.
- Absent marrow iron in the presence of marrow hypercellularity is a feature of PV.
- Chromosomes 3 and 1, where the genes for thrombopoietin and its receptor *Mpl,* respectively, are located.
- Very high platelet counts are associated primarily with hemorrhage due to acquired von Willebrand disease!!! This can be identified by a reduction in ristocetin cofactor activity. In this situation, aspirin could promote hemorrhage. Bleeding in this situation usually responds to e-aminocaproic acid, which can be given prophylactically before and after elective surgery.
- Hodgkin's disease is more common in whites than in blacks and more common in males than in females.
- Patients in the younger age groups diagnosed in the United States largely have the nodular sclerosing subtype of Hodgkin's disease.

- Elderly patients, patients infected with HIV, and patients in Third World countries more commonly have mixed-cellularity Hodgkin's disease or lymphocyte-depleted Hodgkin's disease.
- Non-Hodgkin's lymphomas are more frequent in the elderly and more frequent in men.
- Lymphoplasmacytic lymphoma is associated with Hepatitis-C virus.
- HHV-8 is associated with multicentric castleman's disease.
- MALT lymphomas of the skin may be related to *Borrelia* sp. infections, those of the eyes to *Chlamydophila psittaci*, and those of the small intestine to *Campylobacter jejuni*.
- Many lymphomas contain balanced chromosomal translocations involving the antigen receptor genes; immunoglobulin genes on chromosomes 2, 14, and 22 in B cells; and T cell antigen receptor genes on chromosomes 7 and 14 in T cells.
- In the case of diffuse large B cell lymphoma, the translocation t(14;18) occurs in ~ 30% of patients and leads to overexpression of the *BCL-2* gene found on chromosome 18. Some other patients without the translocation also overexpress the BCL-2 protein.
- In typical B cell CLL, trisomy 12 conveys a poorer prognosis.
- In childhood ALL, hyperdiploidy has been shown to have a favorable prognosis.
- Rai system and Binet system are used to grade lymphoid malignancies.
- ZAP-70 cytoplasmic expression and CD-38 expression shows a poor prognosis in lymphocytic leukemias.
- The prognosis of patients with Non-Hodgkin's lymphoma is best assigned using the International Prognostic Index (IPI)
- The most common treatments for patients with typical B cell CLL/small lymphocytic lymphoma have been chlorambucil or fludarabine, alone or in combination. Bendamustine, an alkylating agent structurally related to nitrogen mustard, is highly effective and is vying with fludarabine as the primary treatment of choice. Alemtuzumab (anti-CD52) is an antibody with activity in the disease, but it kills both B and T cells and is associated with more immunecompromise than rituximab.
- At least two genetic forms of gastric MALT exist: one (accounting for about 50% of cases) characterized by t(11;18)(q21;q21) that juxtaposes the amino terminal of the *API2* gene with the carboxy terminal of the *MALT1* gene creating an API2/MALT1 fusion product, and the other characterized by multiple sites of genetic instability including trisomies of chromosomes 3, 7, 12, and 18.
- t(11;18)-negative MALT lymphomas often acquire *BCL6* mutations and progress to aggressive histology lymphoma.
- An intensive combination chemotherapy regimen originally used in the treatment of acute leukemia, HyperC-VAD (cyclophosphamide, vincristine, doxorubicin, dexamethasone, cytarabine, and methotrexate), in combination with rituximab, seems to be associated with better response rates—particularly in younger patients. Alternating two regimens, HyperC-VAD with rituximab added (R-HyperC-VAD) and rituximab plus high-dose methotrexate and cytarabine can achieve complete responses in > 80% of patients and 8-year survival of 56%, comparable to regimens employing high-dose therapy and autologous hematopoietic stem cell transplantation. Bortezomib, temsirolimus, and bendamustine are single agents that induce transient partial responses in a minority of patients and are being added to primary combinations.
- Confirmation of B cell immunophenotype and the existence of the t(14;18) and abnormal expression of BCL-2 protein are confirmatory.
- Follicular lymphoma is one of the malignancies most responsive to chemotherapy and radiotherapy. In addition, tumors in as many as 25% of the patients undergo spontaneous regression—usually transient—without therapy. In an asymptomatic patient, no initial treatment and watchful waiting can be an appropriate management strategy and is particularly likely to be adopted for older patients with advanced-stage disease.
- For patients who do require treatment, single-agent chlorambucil or cyclophosphamide or combination chemotherapy with CVP or CHOP are most frequently used.
- Patients with follicular lymphoma have a high rate of histologic transformation to diffuse large B cell lymphoma (5–7% per year). This is recognized about 40% of the time during the course of the illness by repeat biopsy and is present in almost all patients at autopsy.

- Diffuse large B cell lymphoma is the most common type of Non-Hodgkin's lymphoma, representing approximately one-third of all cases.
- Patients whose tumors overexpress the BCL-2 protein might be more likely to relapse than others.
- Patients with prominent mediastinal involvement are sometimes diagnosed as a separate subgroup having primary mediastinal diffuse large B cell lymphoma. This latter group of patients has a younger median age (i.e. 37 years) and a female predominance (66%).
- Other unusual subtypes of diffuse large B cell lymphoma such as pleural effusion lymphoma and intravascular lymphoma have been difficult to diagnose and associated with a very poor prognosis.
- Three distinct clinical forms of Burkitt's lymphoma are recognized; endemic, sporadic, and immunodeficiency-associated.
- This is the most rapidly progressive human tumor, and any delay in initiating therapy can adversely affect the patient's prognosis.
- Treatment of Burkitt's lymphoma in both children and adults should begin within 48 hours of diagnosis and involves the use of intensive combination chemotherapy regimens incorporating high doses of cyclophosphamide. Prophylactic therapy to the CNS is mandatory.
- Hairy cell leukemia: The malignant cells appear to have 'hairy' projections on light and electron microscopy and show a characteristic staining pattern with tartrate-resistant acid phosphatase. Patients with this disorder are prone to unusual infections, including infection by *Mycobacterium avium intracellulare*, and to vasculitic syndromes. Hairy cell leukemia is responsive to chemotherapy with interferon α, pentostatin, or cladribine, with the latter being the usually preferred treatment. Clinical complete remissions with cladribine occur in the majority of patients, and long-term disease-free survival is frequent.
- Adult T cell lymphoma/leukemia: Diagnosis is made when an expert hematopathologist recognizes the typical morphologic picture, a T cell immunophenotype (i.e. CD4 positive), and the presence in serum of antibodies to HTLV-I. Examination of the peripheral blood will usually reveal characteristic, pleomorphic abnormal CD4-positive cells with indented nuclei, which have been called 'flower' cells. Most patients present with an aggressive disease manifested by lymphadenopathy, hepatosplenomegaly, skin infiltration, pulmonary infiltrates, hypercalcemia, lytic bone lesions, and elevated LDH levels and the median survival of patients is about 7 months. A small phase II study reported a high response rate with interferon plus zidovudine and arsenic trioxide.
- Anaplastic Large T/Null Cell Lymphoma: Expresses CD30 (Ki-1) antigen, shows t(2;5), and also overexpression of the anaplastic lymphoma kinase (ALK) protein. ALK also seen in non small cell carcinoma of the lung and neuroblastoma. So crizotinib (ALK blocker) is used to treat non small cell carcinoma and is undergoing trials for the other tumors. Surprisingly, given the anaplastic appearance, this disorder has the best survival rate of any aggressive lymphoma. The 5-year survival is > 75%. While traditional prognostic factors such as the IPI predict treatment outcome, overexpression of the ALK protein is an important prognostic factor, with patients overexpressing this protein having a superior treatment outcome. The ALK inhibitor crizotinib appears highly active as well.
- *Extranodal T/NK cell lymphoma of nasal type* has also been called *angiocentric lymphoma* and was previously termed *lethal midline granuloma*. This disorder is more frequent in Asia and South America than in the United States and Europe. EBV is thought to play an etiologic role. Prognosis is poor.
- *Enteropathy-type intestinal T cell lymphoma* is a rare disorder that occurs in patients with untreated gluten-sensitive enteropathy. Patients are frequently wasted and sometimes present with intestinal perforation. The prognosis is poor.
- The development of the hemophagocytic syndrome (profound anemia, ingestion of erythrocytes by monocytes and macrophages) in the course of any peripheral T cell lymphoma is generally associated with a fatal outcome.
- Subdiaphragmatic presentation of Hodgkin's disease is unusual and more common in older males.
- Rarely, the fevers persist for days to weeks, followed by afebrile intervals and then recurrence of the fever. This pattern is known as *Pel-Ebstein fever*.
- The most popular chemotherapy regimens used in Hodgkin's disease include doxorubicin, bleomycin, vinblastine, and dacarbazine (ABVD) and mechlorethamine (blisters), vincristine (neurotoxicity but BM sparing

like bleomycin and asparaginase {VAB}), procarbazine (disulfiram reaction, MAO inhibition producing cheese reaction, peripheral neuropathy), and prednisone (MOPP), or combinations of the drugs in these two regimens.

- Today, most patients in the United States receive ABVD, but a weekly chemotherapy regimen administered for 12 weeks called *Stanford V* is becoming increasingly popular, but includes radiation therapy, which has been associated with life-threatening late toxicities such as premature coronary artery disease and second solid tumors.
- In Europe, a high-dose regimen called *BEACOPP* incorporating alkylating agents has become popular and might have a better response rate in very high-risk patients.
- Lhermitte's syndrome occurs in about 15% of patients who receive thoracic radiotherapy. This syndrome is manifested by an 'electric shock' sensation into the lower extremities on flexion of the neck.
- Specific conditions that can be confused with lymphoma include *Castleman's disease*, which can present with localized or disseminated lymphadenopathy; some patients have systemic symptoms. The disseminated form is often accompanied by anemia and polyclonal hypergammaglobulinemia, and the condition has been associated with overproduction of interleukin 6, possibly produced by human herpesvirus 8.
- *Sinus histiocytosis with massive lymphadenopathy* (*Rosai-Dorfman's disease*) usually presents with bulky lymphadenopathy in children or young adults. The disease is usually nonprogressive and self-limited, but patients can manifest autoimmune hemolytic anemia.
- *Lymphomatoid papulosis* is a cutaneous lymphoproliferative disorder that is often confused with anaplastic large cell lymphoma involving the skin. The cells of lymphomatoid papulosis are similar to those seen in lymphoma and stain for CD30. But the disease is benign. Misdiagnosis is a serious mistake.
- Certain syndromes with somatic cell chromosome aneuploidy, such as trisomy 21 noted in Down syndrome, are associated with an increased incidence of AML. Inherited diseases with defective DNA repair, e.g. Fanconi anemia, Bloom syndrome, and ataxia-telangiectasia, are also associated with AML.
- Congenital neutropenia (Kostmann syndrome) is a disease with mutations in the granulocyte colony-stimulating factor (G-CSF) receptor and, often, neutrophil elastase that may evolve into AML. Myeloproliferative syndromes may also evolve into AML.
- Germ-line mutations of CCAAT/enhancer-binding protein α (*CEBPA*), runt-related transcription factor 1 (*RUNX1*), and tumor protein p53 (*TP53*) have also been associated with a higher predisposition to AML in some series.
- Anticancer drugs are the leading cause of therapy-associated AML. Alkylating agent–associated leukemias occur on average 4–6 years after exposure, and affected individuals have aberrations in chromosomes 5 and 7. Topoisomerase II inhibitor–associated leukemias occur 1–3 years after exposure, and affected individuals often have aberrations involving chromosome 11q23.
- Chloramphenicol, phenylbutazone, and, less commonly, chloroquine and methoxypsoralen can result in bone marrow failure that may evolve into AML.
- M6: Erythroleukemia (DiGuglielmo's disease)
- AML with minimal differentiation that is characterized by immature morphology and no lineage-specific cytochemical reactions may be diagnosed by flow-cytometric demonstration of the myeloid-specific antigens cluster designation (CD) 13 and/or 117. Similarly, acute megakaryoblastic leukemia can often be diagnosed only by expression of the platelet-specific antigens CD41 and/or CD61.

Lymphomas and Leukemias

Pre b ALL	CD19, 20+, TdT + No IgM
Pre T ALL	CD1, 2, 5, 7+ CD3, 4, 8+/- TdT+
CLL	CD23, 5+, smudge cells, AIHA, can turn into DLBCL (Richter syndrome)
Follicular	CD 10, 19, 20+ t(14;18) Bcl2+ CD5-
Mantle	CD5+ CD23- t(11;14) lymphomatoid polyposis +
Marginal	CD20+ t(11;18) TRAP+ may occur in Sjogren

Contd...

Contd...

MALToma	Similar to above
DLBCL	Bcl6+ CD20+ vesicular appearance of nucleus with prominent nucleoli and marginated chromatin
Adult T cell	Clover leaf or flower shaped nucleus
Anaplastic large cell	CD30+, ALK+, hallmark cells
Nodular sclerosis HL	Female predominance, good prognosis, lacunar RS cell
Mixed cellularity HL	M/c in India, EBV+ mononuclear variant
Lymphocyte rich HL	EBV+
Lymphocyte depleted HL	Reticular variant, HIV associated
Lymphocyte predominant HL	CD20, 45+ CD15, 30- Pop corn variant, BCl6+
Extranodal T cell	Angiocentric lymphoma, male predominance
AML Mo	MPO-
M1	MPO+
M2	t(8;21) chloroma, good prognosis
M3	T(15;17) DIC+
M4	Inv16
M5	T(9;11)
M6	DiGuglielmo's disease
M7	Down syndrome+
MULTIPLE MYELOMA	Normal ALP, increased ESR, Proximal RTA+, decreased AG, gamma globinemia+

BCL6

- Burkitt's
- DLBCL
- Lymphocyte predominant HL

TRAP

- Hairy cell
- Marginal zone
- Gaucher's
- Osteoclastoma/osteoporosis
- Metastatic bone disease
- HIV encephalopathy

PLASMA CELL DISORDER

MGUS

- BM plasma cell < 10%
- Sr. monoclonal protein < 3g/dL
- No end organ damage

Smoldering myeloma

- BM plasma cell 10–30%
- IgG > 3.4 or IgA > 2
- No end organ damage

Indolent Myeloma

- BM plasma cell > 30
- IgG > 3.5 IgA > 2
- Lytic lesions < 3
- No renal failure
- With renal failure and end organ damage = Multiple myeloma

Erythrocytosis in

- RCC
- VHL syndrome
- Adrenal adenoma
- Pheochromocytoma
- Uterine leiomyoma
- Hepatoma
- Meningioma

Bernard-Soulier syndrome	Glanzmann thrombesthenia
• AR	• AR
• GpIb/IX	• Gp IIb/IIIa
• Decreased adhesion	• Decreased aggregation
• No aggregation with ristocetin	• Increased aggregation with ristocetin
• Large platelets	• Normal size

CHAPTER 8

Pharmacology

GENERAL PHARMACOLOGY—CONCEPTS AND FACTS

Bioavailability is the fraction of administered drug that reaches the systemic circulation. Bioavailability is expressed as the fraction of administered drug that gains access to the systemic circulation in a chemically unchanged form. For example, if 100 mg of a drug are administered orally and 70 mg of this drug are absorbed unchanged, the bioavailability is 0.7 or seventy percent.

- Factors that influence bioavailability:
  - First-pass hepatic metabolism
  - Solubility of the drug
  - Chemical instability
  - Nature of the drug formulation (Drug absorption may be altered by factors unrelated to the chemistry of the drug. For example, particle size, salt form, crystal polymorphism, enteric coatings and the presence of excipients (such as binders and dispersing agents) can influence the ease of dissolution and, therefore, alter the rate of absorption.)
- Two related drugs are bioequivalent if they show comparable bioavailability and similar times to achieve peak blood concentrations. Two related drugs with a significant difference in bioavailability are said to be bioinequivalent.
- Two similar drugs are therapeutically equivalent if they have comparable efficacy and safety. [Note: Clinical effectiveness often depends on both the maximum serum drug concentrations and on the time required (after administration) to reach peak concentration. Therefore, two drugs that are bioequivalent may not be therapeutically equivalent.]
- Drug distribution is the process by which a drug reversibly leaves the bloodstream and enters the interstitium (extracellular fluid) and/or the cells of the tissues. The delivery of a drug from the plasma to the interstitium primarily depends on blood flow, capillary permeability, the degree of binding of the drug to plasma and tissue proteins, and the relative hydrophobicity of the drug.
- The major factor influencing the hydrophobic drug's distribution is the blood flow to the area.
- Plasma albumin is the major drug-binding protein and may act as a drug reservoir; that is, as the concentration of the free drug decreases due to elimination by metabolism or excretion, the bound drug dissociates from the protein. This maintains the free-drug concentration as a constant fraction of the total drug in the plasma.
- The volume of distribution is a hypothetical volume of fluid into which a drug is dispersed. Although the volume of distribution has no physiologic or physical basis, it is sometimes useful to compare the distribution of a drug with the volumes of the water compartments in the body.
- The volume into which drugs distribute is called the apparent volume of distribution, or V_d. Another useful way to think of this constant is as the partition coefficient of a drug between the plasma and the rest of the body.
- If the V_d for a drug is large, most of the drug is in the extraplasmic space and is unavailable to the excretory organs. Therefore, any factor that increases the volume of distribution can lead to an increase in the half-life and extend the duration of action of the drug. [Note: An exceptionally large V_d indicates considerable sequestration of the drug in some organ or compartment.]

- Albumin has the strongest affinities for anionic drugs (weak acids) and hydrophobic drugs. Most hydrophilic drugs and neutral drugs do not bind to albumin. [Note: Many drugs are hydrophobic by design, because this property permits absorption after oral administration.]
- Class I drugs: If the dose of drug is less than the binding capacity of albumin, then the dose/capacity ratio is low.
- Class II drugs: These drugs are given in doses that greatly exceed the number of albumin binding sites.
- Clinical importance of drug displacement: This assignment of drug classification assumes importance when a patient taking a Class I drug, such as warfarin, is given a Class II drug, such as a sulfonamide antibiotic. Warfarin is highly bound to albumin, and only a small fraction is free. This means that most of the drug is sequestered on albumin and is inert in terms of exerting pharmacologic actions. If a sulfonamide is administered, it displaces warfarin from albumin, leading to a rapid increase in the concentration of free warfarin in plasma, because almost 100 percent is now free, compared with the initial small percentage. [Note: The increase in warfarin concentration may lead to increased therapeutic effects, as well as increased toxic effects, such as bleeding.
- Cytochrome P450, designated as CYP, is composed of many families of heme-containing isozymes that are located in most cells but are primarily found in the liver and GI tract. The family name is indicated by an arabic number followed by a capital letter for the subfamily (for example, CYP3A). Another number is added to indicate the specific isozyme (CYP3A4).
- CYP2D6, in particular, has been shown to exhibit genetic polymorphism.
- Some individuals, e.g. obtain no benefit from the opioid analgesic codeine because they lack the enzyme that O-demethylates and activates the drug. This reaction is CYP2D6-dependent.
- Certain drugs, most notably phenobarbital, rifampin, and carbamazepine, are capable of increasing the synthesis of one or more CYP isozymes. This results in increased biotransformations of drugs and can lead to significant decreases in plasma concentrations of drugs metabolized by these CYP isozymes, as measured by AUC, with concurrent loss of pharmacologic effect. For example, rifampin, an antituberculosis drug significantly decreases the plasma concentrations of human immunodeficiency virus (HIV) protease inhibitors, diminishing their ability to suppress HIV virion maturation.
- In addition to drugs, natural substances and pollutants can also induce CYP isozymes. For example, polycyclic aromatic hydrocarbons (found as air pollutants) can induce CYP1A. This has implications for certain drugs; e.g. amitriptyline and warfarin are metabolized by P4501A2. Polycyclic hydrocarbons induce P4501A2, which decreases the therapeutic concentrations of these agents.
- The most common form of inhibition is through competition for the same isozyme. Some drugs, however, are capable of inhibiting reactions for which they are not substrates (e.g. ketoconazole), leading to drug interactions.
- Numerous drugs have been shown to inhibit one or more of the CYP-dependent biotransformation pathways of warfarin. For example, omeprazole is a potent inhibitor of three of the CYP isozymes responsible for warfarin metabolism.
- Phase I reactions not involving the P450 system: These include amine oxidation (e.g. oxidation of catecholamines or histamine), alcohol dehydrogenation (e.g. ethanol oxidation), esterases (e.g. metabolism of pravastatin in liver), and hydrolysis (e.g. of procaine).
- A notable exception is morphine-6-glucuronide, which is more potent than morphine.
- Glucuronidation is the most common and the most important conjugation reaction. Neonates are deficient in this conjugating system, making them particularly vulnerable to drugs such as chloramphenicol, which is inactivated by the addition of glucuronic acid.
- Not all drugs undergo Phase I and II reactions in that order. For example, isoniazid is first acetylated (a Phase II reaction) and then hydrolyzed to isonicotinic acid (a Phase I reaction).
- Removal of a drug from the body occurs via a number of routes, the most important being through the kidney into the urine. Other routes include the bile, intestine, lung, or milk in nursing mothers.
- As a general rule, weak acids can be eliminated by alkalinization of the urine, whereas elimination of weak bases may be increased by acidification of the urine.
- For example, a patient presenting with phenobarbital (weak acid) overdose can be given bicarbonate, which alkalinizes the urine and keeps the drug ionized, thereby decreasing its reabsorption. If overdose is with a weak

base, such as cocaine, acidification of the urine with NH_4Cl leads to protonation of the drug and an increase in its clearance.

- The steady-state plasma concentration is directly proportional to the infusion rate. For example, if the infusion rate is doubled, the plasma concentration ultimately achieved at the steady state is doubled.
- Thus, fifty percent of the final steady-state concentration of drug is observed after the time elapsed since the infusion, t, is equal to $t_{1/2}$, where $t_{1/2}$ (or half-life) is the time required for the drug concentration to change by fifty percent. For convenience, therefore, one can assume that a drug will reach steady-state in about four half-lives.
- As in the case for IV infusion, ninety percent of the steady-state value is achieved in 3.3 times $t_{1/2}$.
- When repeated administration of a drug results in a diminished effect, the phenomenon is called tachyphylaxis.
- Potency, a measure of the amount of drug necessary to produce an effect of a given magnitude.
- Efficacy is the ability of a drug to illicit a physiologic response when it interacts with a receptor. Efficacy is dependent on the number of drug–receptor complexes formed and the efficiency of the coupling of receptor activation to cellular responses.
- A fundamental principle of pharmacodynamics is that drugs only modify underlying biochemical and physiological processes; they do not create effects *de novo*.
- Pharmacology defines a receptor as any biologic molecule to which a drug binds and produces a measurable response. Thus, enzymes and structural proteins can be considered to be pharmacologic receptors. However, the richest sources of therapeutically exploitable pharmacologic receptors are proteins that are responsible for transducing extracellular signals into intracellular responses.
- The most common enzyme-linked receptors (epidermal growth factor, platelet-derived growth factor, atrial natriuretic peptide, insulin, and others) are those that have a tyrosine kinase activity as part of their structure.
- Due to amplification, only a fraction of the total receptors for a specific ligand may need to be occupied to elicit a maximal response from a cell. Systems that exhibit this behavior are said to have spare receptors. Spare receptors are exhibited by insulin receptors, where it has been estimated that 99 percent of the receptors are 'spare'.
- When repeated administration of a drug results in a diminished effect, the phenomenon is called tachyphylaxis.
- The relationship between dose and response is a continuous one, and it can be mathematically described for many systems by application of the law of mass action. The response is a graded effect, meaning that the response is continuous and gradual. This contrasts with a quantal response, which describes an all-or-nothing response. A graph of this relationship is known as a graded dose–response curve.
- Rectangular hyperbola- dose response curve.
  Sigmoidal- log dose response curve.
- If a drug binds to a receptor and produces a biologic response that mimics the response to the endogenous ligand, it is known as an agonist.
- Antagonists are drugs that decrease the actions of another drug or endogenous ligand. Antagonists, however, have no intrinsic activity and, therefore, produce no effect by themselves. Although antagonists have no intrinsic activity, they are able to bind avidly to target receptors because they possess strong affinity.
- A unique feature of a partial agonist is that, under appropriate conditions, these drugs may act as an antagonist of a full agonist.
- EC_{50} = drug dose that shows fifty percent of maximal response is the potency of the drug.
- Another important dose–response relationship is that of the influence of the magnitude of the dose on the proportion of a population that responds. These responses are known as quantal responses, because, for any individual, the effect either occurs or it does not.
- The therapeutic index of a drug is the ratio of the dose that produces toxicity to the dose that produces a clinically desired or effective response in a population of individuals.
- Most drugs have molecular weights between 100 and 1000. The lower limit of this narrow range is probably set by the requirements for specificity of action. The upper limit in molecular weight is determined primarily by the requirement that drugs must be able to move within the body (e.g. from the site of administration to the site of action).

- The specific nature of a particular drug-receptor bond is of less practical importance than the fact that drugs that bind through weak bonds to their receptors are generally more selective than drugs that bind by means of very strong bonds. This is because weak bonds require a very precise fit of the drug to its receptor if an interaction is to occur. Only a few receptor types are likely to provide such a precise fit for a particular drug structure.
- Rational design of drugs implies the ability to predict the appropriate molecular structure of a drug on the basis of information about its biologic receptor.
- Thus, pindolol, a β-adrenoceptor partial agonist, may act either as an agonist (if no full agonist is present) or as an antagonist (if a full agonist such as epinephrine is present). Intrinsic efficacy is independent of affinity for the receptor.
- In some cases, an inactive precursor chemical that is readily absorbed and distributed must be administered and then converted to the active drug by biologic processes—inside the body. Such a precursor chemical is called a **prodrug.**
- Lipid diffusion is the most important limiting factor for drug permeation because of the large number of lipid barriers that separate the compartments of the body. Because these lipid barriers separate aqueous compartments, the lipid: aqueous partition coefficient of a drug determines how readily the molecule moves between aqueous and lipid media.
- More of a weak acid will be in the lipid-soluble form at acid pH, whereas more of a basic drug will be in the lipid-soluble form at alkaline pH.
- Thus, weak acids are usually excreted faster in alkaline urine; weak bases are usually excreted faster in acidic urine.
- Therefore, primary, secondary, and tertiary amines may undergo reversible protonation and vary their lipid solubility with pH, but quaternary amines are always in the poorly lipid-soluble charged form.
- Now, receptors are being discovered by predicted structure or sequence homology to other (known) receptors, and drugs that bind to them are developed later using chemical screening methods. This effort has revealed, for many known drugs, a larger diversity of receptors than previously anticipated. It has also identified a number of **'orphan' receptors,** so-called because their ligands are presently unknown, which may prove to be useful targets for the development of new drugs.
- The transduction process that links drug occupancy of receptors and pharmacologic response is often termed **coupling.**
- Protamine, a protein that is positively charged at physiologic pH, can be used clinically to counteract the effects of heparin, an anticoagulant that is negatively charged. In this case, one drug acts as a **chemical antagonist** of the other simply by ionic binding that makes the other drug unavailable for interactions with proteins involved in blood clotting.
- Verapamil inhibits voltage-gated calcium channels that are present in the heart and in vascular smooth muscle, producing antiarrhythmic effects and reducing blood pressure.
- Almost all second messenger signaling involves reversible phosphorylation, which performs two principal functions in signaling: amplification and flexible regulation.
- The clinical effectiveness of a drug depends not on its potency (EC_{50}), but on its maximal efficacy. In deciding which of two drugs to administer to a patient, the prescriber must usually consider their relative effectiveness rather than their relative potency. Pharmacologic potency can largely determine the administered dose of the chosen drug.
- Steep dose-response curves in patients can result from cooperative interactions of several different actions of a drug (e.g. effects on brain, heart, and peripheral vessels, all contributing to lowering of blood pressure).
- Some of these difficulties may be avoided by determining the dose of drug required to produce a specified magnitude of effect in a large number of individual patients or experimental animals and plotting the cumulative frequency distribution of responders versus the log dose. The specified quantal effect may be chosen on the basis of clinical relevance (e.g. relief of headache) or for preservation of safety of experimental subjects (e.g. using low doses of a cardiac stimulant and specifying an increase in heart rate of 20 bpm as the quantal effect), or it may be an inherently quantal event (e.g. death of an experimental animal).

- For most drugs, the doses required to produce a specified quantal effect in individuals are lognormally distributed; that is, a frequency distribution of such responses plotted against the log of the dose produces a gaussian normal curve of variation. When these responses are summated, the resulting cumulative frequency distribution constitutes a quantal dose-effect curve (or dose-percent curve) of the proportion or percentage of individuals who exhibit the effect plotted as a function of log dose.
- The quantal dose-effect curve is often characterized by stating the **median effective dose (ED_{50}),** which is the dose at which 50% of individuals exhibit the specified quantal effect. (Note that the abbreviation ED_{50} has a different meaning in this context from its meaning in relation to graded dose-effect curves, described in previous text). Similarly, the dose required to produce a particular toxic effect in 50% of animals is called the **median toxic dose (TD_{50}).** If the toxic effect is death of the animal, a **median lethal dose (LD_{50})** may be experimentally defined.
- One can obtain a valuable index of the selectivity of a drug's action by comparing its ED_{50}s for two different quantal effects in a population (e.g. cough suppression versus sedation for opioid drugs).
- Quantal dose-effect curves may also be used to generate information regarding the margin of safety to be expected from a particular drug used to produce a specified effect. One measure, which relates the dose of a drug required to produce a desired effect to that which produces an undesired effect, is the **therapeutic index.** In animal studies, the therapeutic index is usually defined as the ratio of the TD_{50} to the ED_{50} for some therapeutically relevant effect.
- The clinically acceptable risk of toxicity depends critically on the severity of the disease being treated. For example, the dose range that provides relief from an ordinary headache in the majority of patients should be very much lower than the dose range that produces serious toxicity, even if the toxicity occurs in a small minority of patients. However, for treatment of a lethal disease such as Hodgkin's lymphoma, the acceptable difference between therapeutic and toxic doses may be smaller.
- When responsiveness diminishes rapidly after administration of a drug, the response is said to be subject to **tachyphylaxis.**
- Saralasin, a weak partial agonist at angiotensin II receptors, lowers blood pressure in patients with hypertension caused by increased angiotensin II production and raises blood pressure in patients who produce normal amounts of angiotensin.
- Thus, the propensity of drugs to bind to different classes of receptor sites is not only a potentially vexing problem in treating patients, it also presents a continuing challenge to pharmacology and an opportunity for developing new and more useful drugs.
- Pharmacodynamics governs the concentration-effect part of the interaction, whereas pharmacokinetics deals with the dose-concentration part (Holford and Sheiner, 1981).
- The two basic parameters are **clearance,** the measure of the ability of the body to eliminate the drug; and **volume of distribution,** the measure of the apparent space in the body available to contain the drug.
- When clearance is first-order, rate of elimination can be estimated by calculating the **Area Under the Curve (AUC)** of the time-concentration profile after a dose.
- $t1/2 = 0.7 \times V_d/CL$
- Inhibition of P-glycoprotein and gut wall metabolism, e.g. by grapefruit juice, may be associated with substantially increased drug absorption.
- Extraction ratio (ER) is the ratio of clearance in liver to the liver blood flow. (e.g. 0.5 is the extraction ratio when 50% of the drug is extracted when it flows through the liver. That is, say, the clearance is 100 ml per min and the liver blood flow is 200 ml per min then the extraction ratio (ER) is 0.5)
- They denote the fraction of drug absorbed from the gut as "f".

  'F' is the systemic bioavailability.

  Then, $F = f \times (1–ER)$

  (i.e. 1–ER will give you fraction left after liver metabolism. That multiplied with the fraction left after gut absorption will give you the fraction of the drug that is bioavailable. For example, say, 50% is absorbed and 50% of the remaining drug is metabolized then the bioavailability is 25%. ($0.5 \times 0.5 = 0.25 = 25\%$)
- The mechanism of drug absorption is said to be zero-order when the rate is independent of the amount of drug remaining in the gut, e.g. when it is determined by the rate of gastric emptying or by a controlled-release

drug formulation. In contrast, when the full dose is dissolved in gastrointestinal fluids, the rate of absorption is usually proportional to the gastrointestinal concentration and is said to be first-order.

- Lidocaine and verapamil are both used to treat cardiac arrhythmias and have bioavailability less than 40%, but lidocaine is never given orally because its metabolites are believed to contribute to central nervous system toxicity. Other drugs that are highly extracted by the liver include isoniazid, morphine, propranolol, verapamil, and several tricyclic antidepressants.
- Drugs that are poorly extracted by the liver include chlorpropamide, diazepam, phenytoin, theophylline, tolbutamide, and warfarin.
- The renal toxicity of aminoglycoside antibiotics (e.g. gentamicin) is greater when administered as a constant infusion than with intermittent dosing. It is the accumulation of aminoglycoside in the renal cortex that is thought to cause renal damage.
- Thus, if the desired target concentration is known, the clearance in that patient will determine the dosing rate.
- Note that the steady-state concentration achieved by continuous infusion or the *average* concentration following intermittent dosing depends only on clearance. The volume of distribution and the half-life need not be known in order to determine the average plasma concentration expected from a given dosing rate or to predict the dosing rate for a desired target concentration.
- Recognition of the essential role of concentration in linking pharmacokinetics and pharmacodynamics leads naturally to the target concentration strategy. Pharmacodynamic principles can be used to predict the concentration required to achieve a particular degree of therapeutic effect. This target concentration can then be achieved by using pharmacokinetic principles to arrive at a suitable dosing regimen (Holford, 1999). The target concentration strategy is a process for optimizing the dose in an individual on the basis of a measured surrogate response such as drug concentration.
- Drugs such as phenytoin, salicylates, and disopyramide are extensively bound to plasma albumin.
- α_1-Acid glycoprotein is an important binding protein with binding sites for drugs such as quinidine, lidocaine, and propranolol.
- When drug interactions associated with protein binding displacement and clinically important effects have been studied, it has been found that the displacing drug is also an inhibitor of clearance, and it is the change in *clearance* of the *unbound* drug that is the relevant mechanism explaining the interaction.
- Clearance is readily estimated from the dosing rate (in so much mg per min) and mean steady-state concentration (mg per ml).

  Remember?? Dosing rate = Rate of elimination

  And also we have, Rate of elimination = Clearance × Concentration

  So we can calculate the Dosing rate as Clearance × Target concentration (TC is the concentration you are trying to achieve). So we can easily calculate clearance from the Rate of elimination (= Dosing rate) and the steady state concentration (= Target concentration)
- Phase I reactions usually convert the parent drug to a more polar metabolite by introducing or unmasking a functional group (–OH, $-NH_2$, –SH).
- A great variety of drugs undergo the sequential biotransformation reactions, although in some instances the parent drug may already possess a functional group that may form a conjugate directly. For example, the hydrazide moiety of isoniazid is known to form an *N*-acetyl conjugate in a phase II reaction. This conjugate is then a substrate for a phase I type reaction, namely, hydrolysis to isonicotinic acid Thus, phase II reactions may actually precede phase I reactions.
- Some orally administered drugs (e.g. clonazepam, chlorpromazine, cyclosporine) are more extensively metabolized in the intestine than in the liver, whereas others (e.g. midazolam) undergo significant (50%) intestinal metabolism.
- Microsomes contain the important class of enzymes known as the **mixed function oxidases** (MFOs), or **monooxygenases.** The activity of these enzymes requires both a reducing agent (nicotinamide adenine dinucleotide phosphate [NADPH]) and molecular oxygen; in a typical reaction, one molecule of oxygen is consumed (reduced) per substrate molecule, with one oxygen atom appearing in the product and the other in the form of water.

- A Pregnane X Receptor (PXR), a member of the steroid-retinoid-thyroid hormone receptor family, has recently been shown to mediate CYP3A induction by various chemicals (dexamethasone, rifampin, mifepristone, phenobarbital, atorvastatin, and hyperforin, a constituent of St. John's wort) in the liver and intestinal mucosa. A similar receptor, the Constitutive Androstane Receptor (CAR) has been identified for the relatively large and structurally diverse phenobarbital class of inducers of CYP2B6, CYP2C9 and CYP3A4.
- Peroxisome proliferator receptor α (PPARα) is yet another nuclear receptor highly expressed in liver and kidneys, which uses lipid-lowering drugs (e.g. fenofibrate and gemfibrozil) as ligands.
- Barbiturate secobarbital is found to inactivate CYP2B1 by modification of *both* its heme and protein moieties.
- Common types of conjugation are glucuronidation, acetylation, glycine conjugation, sulfation, glutathione conjugation, methylation and water conjugation.
- Furthermore, sulfation is known to activate the orally active prodrug minoxidil into a very efficacious vasodilator, and morphine-6-glucuronide is more potent than morphine itself.
- Succinylcholine is metabolized only half as rapidly in persons with genetically determined defects in pseudocholinesterase as in persons with normally functioning pseudocholinesterase.
- The slow acetylator phenotype is also associated with a higher incidence of drug-induced autoimmune disorders and bicyclic aromatic amine-induced bladder cancer.
- **Debrisoquin-sparteine oxidation** type of polymorphism, which apparently occurs in 3–10% of whites and is inherited as an autosomal recessive trait. In affected individuals, the **CYP2D6**-dependent oxidations of debrisoquin and other drugs are impaired.
- **Ultrarapid metabolism** of relevant drugs due to the presence of 2D6 allelic variants with up to 13 gene copies in tandem, require twofold to threefold higher daily doses of nortriptyline (a 2D6 substrate) to achieve therapeutic plasma levels. Conversely, in these ultrarapid-metabolizing populations, the prodrug codeine (another 2D6 substrate) is metabolized much faster to morphine, often resulting in undesirable adverse effects of morphine, such as abdominal pain.
- Finally, the release of inflammatory mediators, cytokines, and nitric oxide associated with bacterial or viral infections, cancer, or inflammation are known to impair drug metabolism by inactivating P450s and enhancing their degradation.
- Ames test, tests the effects on genetic stability and mutations in bacteria.
- Subject bias effects can be quantitated—and minimized relative to the response measured during active therapy—by the single-blind design.
- Angiogenesis inhibitors such as angiostatin and endostatin were shown to be proteins that were fragments of the endogenous proteins collagen or plasminogen.
- In 2004, bevacizumab (Avastin) became the first antiangiogenesis drug to receive FDA approval. It is intended for combination use with standard chemotherapy for metastatic colon cancer. Approval for other indications as part of combination therapy followed: non-small-cell lung cancer and breast cancer.

Enzyme Inducer

- Barbiturate
- CBZ
- Rifampicin
- Alcohol
- Efavirenz
- Phenytoin
- Griseofulvin
- DDT
- Nevirapine

Enzyme Inhibitor

- Amiodarone
- Azoles
- CCB
- Disulfiram
- Macrolides-erythromycin
- Allopurinol
- Cimetidine
- Cyclosporine
- Fluoroquinolone-cipro
- Omeprazole

- Lansoprazole
- Valproate
- Protease inhibitor

PRE-, PRO-, AND SYMBIOTICS

Probiotics	Flora beneficial in GIT
Prebiotics	Enhance probiotic
Synbiotics	Synergistic with above two

Increased Rennin

- ACE/ARB
- Cirrhosis
- Diuretics
- Renal nerve stimulation
- Sympathetic stimulation
- Upright posture
- Dipyridamol
- Secondary hyperaldosteronism

Decreased Rennin

- Angiotensin 2
- Alpha 2 agonist
- NSAID
- Increased NaCl absorption in macula
- Primary hyperaldosteronism (Conn)
- Vasopressin
- Beta blocker
- Clonidine
- Increased afferent arterial pressure

Decreased ESR

- Sickle cell
- Afibrinogenemia
- Polycythemia
- CCF

Phase I

- P50 oxidation (monooxygenase)
- Deaminase
- Esterase
- Chloroquine
- Fluoxetine
- Dehydrogenase
- Desulfration
- Increased volume of distribution:
- Digoxin

Phase II

- Sulphtransferase
- Acetylase
- Glutathione transferase
- Methylase
- Glucoronyl transferase
- Glycine transferase

Acetylation and SLE *(SHIP)*

- Sulphonamide
- INH
- Hydralazine
- Procainamide

Only biliary excretion

- Erythromycin
- Metronidazole
- Rifampicin
- Azithromycin
- Naficillin
- Tigicyclin

Zero-order kinetics

- Alcohol
- Aspirin
- Hydralazine
- Propranalol
- Phenytoin
- Theophylline
- Tolbutamide
- Cetuximab

Basic Drugs are Excreted Through Breast

Drugs worsening myasthenia gravis

- Quinine
- Beta blocker
- Muscle relaxants
- Penicillamine
- Macrolides
- Aminoglycoside
- $MgSO_4$
- Lithium
- Tetracycline

Difference between tacrolimus and sirolimus

Tacrolimus	More nephro and neurotoxic, alopecia, diarrhea, diabetes
Sirolimus	Increases lipids, decreases platelets

Autonomic receptors action:

Sympathetic

α1 – Pupil dilatation, pilo erection, ejaculation, vasoconstriction
α2 – ↓sympathetic activity, inhibit lipolysis, platelet aggregation, inhibit insulin release
β1 – ↑HR, SBP, ↑Renin
β2 – Bronchodilation, uterine relaxation, bladder relaxation, skeletal muscle potassium uptake(↓K), ↑glucogenesis and glycogenolysis, vasodilation
β3 – Lipolysis

Note:

α1, α2, β1, β2 – Inhibit peristalsis
No β2 antagonist drug used therapeutically.

Parasympathetic

M1 – CNS, Gastric glands, ganglion
M2 – Heart
M3 – Exocrine glands, smooth muscles, endothelium

Eye

α1 - Dilator pupillae
β - Ciliary epithelium
M3 - Sphincter papillae, ciliary muscle

Drugs	Receptors
Adrenaline	α1, α2, β1, β2
Noradrenaline	α1*, α2, β1, β3 (no β2)
Dopamine	D1*, D2, α1, α2, β1 (no β2)
Dobutamine	β1*, β2, α1, α2 (no D)
Isoprenaline	β1*, β2, β3
Fenoldopam	D, α2

Arrhythmia	Mechanism
Atrial fibrillation	Functional re-entry
Atrial flutter	Re-entry in RA
PSVT	Re-entry in AV node
VT and VF in Myocardial Infarction	Functional re-entry
Torsade pointes	EAD

Vaughan William Classification:

Class	Drugs
I a (increases APD)	Procainamide, disopyramide, quinidine
I b	Phenytoin, lidocaine, mexiletine, tocainide
I c	Propafenone, flecainide, encainide, moricizine
II	Propranolol, acebutolol, esmolol
III (increases APD)	Amiodarone, Bretylium, Ibutilide, Sotalol
IV	Verapamil, Diltiazem

Opioid receptors

Opioid agonist—Antagonist:

Opioid	Agonist	Antagonist
Buprenorphine	μ (Partial)	κ
Nalbuphine	κ	μ
Dzocine	κ	μ
Butorphanol	κ	μ (Partial)
Pentazocine	κ	μ (Partial)
Methadone	μ	–

μ: Endorphin:

- Miosis
- Analgesia
- Euphoria
- Muscle rigidity
- Constipation
- Resp depression
- Sedation

Kappa: Dynorphin:

- Dysphoria
- Analgesia
- Diuresis

Delta: Encephalin:

- Spinal analgesia
- NT release

DHFR inhibitors

- Methotrexate
- Pentamidine
- Trimethoprim
- Pyrimethamine
- Proguanil
- Triampterine

Folate Abs inhibitors

- Primidone
- Phenobarbitone
- Septran
- Phenytoin
- Carbamazepine
- Sulfasalazine

Folate synthesis inhibitors:

- PAS
- Sulfonamides
- Dapsone

Protein Synthesis Inhibitors

Aminoglycosides	30s and 50s freezing initiation, misreading mRNA
Tetracyclines	30s inhibit aminoacyl tRNA attachment
Spectinomycin 30s	same mech
Linezolide	23s and 50s inhibit initiation (mutation of 23s)
Chloramphenicol	50s inhibit peptidyl transferase
Cycloheximide	60s
Macrolides	50s inhibit translocation
Streptogramins	50s

Cell Wall

Betalactams	transpeptidase
Vancomycin	transglycolase
Cycloserine	alanine racemase and ligase
Bacitracin	dephosphorylation of bactoprenol
Fesfomycin	Enolpyruvate transferase

Antivirals

Entry – *Enfuvirtide, Docosonol, Palivizumab*

↓

Penetration – *Interferon*

↓

Uncoating – *Amantidine*

↓

Nucleic acid synthesis – *NRTI, NNRTI, Acylovir, Foscarnet*

↓

Late protein synthesis – *Protease inhibitors*

↓

Package and release – *Neuraminidase inhibitors – Zanamivir, Oseltamivir*

Hyperkalemia:

- ACE inhibitors
- Heparin
- Trimethoprim
- Cyclosporine
- NSAIDs
- Potassium-sparing diuretics
- Pentamidine
- Succinyl choline

Hypokalemia:

- Amphotericin B
- Penicillin

- Gentamicin
- Theophylline
- Corticosteroids
- Insulin
- Tetracycline
- Carbenoxolone
- Diuretics

Hyperglycemia:

- Epinephrine
- Corticosteroids
- Diuretics
- Protease inhibitors
- Clozapine
- Beta 2 agonist
- Pot channel opener
- Phenytoin
- INF alpha

Hypoglycemia:

- Beta blocker
- Lithium
- Pentamidine
- Salicylates
- Clofibrate
- Theophylline
- Quinine
- Sulphonamides

Polypeptides:

- Polymyxin B
- Thyroticin
- Colistin
- Bacitracin

Polyenes:

- Amphotericin
- Hamycin
- Nystatin
- Natamycin

Azoles:

- Ketoconazole
- Fluconazole
- Voriconazole
- Itaconazole
- Clotrimazole

Hirsutism:

- Potassium channel opener
- Phenytoin
- Progesterone
- Cyclosporine
- Anabolic steroid
- Danazol

Gynecomastia:

- Digitalis
- Ketoconazole
- Cimetidine
- Ethionamide
- Alpha methyl dopa
- Flutamide
- Cyproterone acetate
- Spironolactone
- Griseofulvin
- Reserpine
- INH
- CCB
- Goserelin

Bone marrow toxicity:

- Chloramphenicol
- Gold
- Phenytoin
- NSAID
- Ziduvudine
- CBZ

- Felbamate
- Colchicines
- Antimetabolites
- Carbimazole
- Trimethadione
- Cytotoxics
- Alkylating agent
- Anthracycline
- Thioamide

Thalidomide—USES:

- AIDS related aphtous ulcers
- Multiple myeloma
- Rheumatoid arthritis
- Bechets
- AIDS related wasting syndrome
- GVH, SLE
- Ankylosing spondylitis
- ENL

Adverse effects—Corticosteroids, sedation, peripheral neuropathy, DVT, constipation

Hand-foot syndrome:

- 5 fluorouracil
- Cytarabine
- Sorafenib
- Cepecitabine
- Doxorubicin
- Sunitinib

Cardiotoxicity:

- Anthracycline
- Bevacizumab
- Taxane
- Transtuzumab
- Imatinid, desatinib

Pulmonary fibrosis:

- Bleomycin
- Mitomycin
- Amiodarone
- Methysergide
- Methotrexate
- Alkylating agents
- Busulfan

BM toxicity:

- Alkylating agents
- Anthracyclines
- Bleomycin
- Vincristine
- Antimetabolites
- Asparaginase
- Gefitinib
- Hormonal agents

Disulfiram reaction:

- Procarbazine
- Cefotetan
- Moxalactam
- Chlorpropamide
- Cefmandole
- Cefoperazone
- Griseofulvin
- Metronidazole

Category	Study
A	No risk
B	Animal study no risk, no human study
C	Animal study risk, no human study
D	Proven risk, benefit at weight risk
X	Risks outweigh benefits

Cell cycle-specific

Antimetabolites	S
Epidophylotoxin	G2S
Taxane	M
Campothecin	S
Vinca alkaloids	M
Ixabepilone	M
Bleomycin	G2
Hydroxyurea	S

Nonspecific

- Alkylating agents
- Platinum compounds
- Antitumor antibodies

Plant origin

- Taxanes
- Podophyllotoxin
- Camptothecin
- Vinca alkaloids

Microtubules

- Vinca alkaloids
- Estramustin
- Taxanes
- Ixabepilone

MDR 1 gene-p glycoprotein efflux

- Anthracycline
- Etoposide
- Vinca alkaloids
- Taxanes

Topoisomerase 1

- Topotecan
- Irinotecan

Topoisomerase 2

- Podophyllotoxin
- Anthracycline

Anaerobes

- Metronidazole
- Meropenem/imipenem
- Ticarcillin/clavulanic acid
- Vancomycin
- Cefoxitin
- Moxifloxacin
- Clindamycin
- Chloramphenicol
- Ampicillin/sulbactam
- Cefotetan
- Cefmetazole

Ribavirin

- RSV
- Adenovirus
- SARS
- Measles
- Lassa virus

Hepatitis B

- Entecavir
- Tenofovir
- Telbivudin
- Adefovir
- Lamivudine
- INF alpha

Aminoglycosides

Streptomycin	maximum neuromuscular blockade, max vestibulotoxic, min nephrotoxic
Max. nephrotoxic	Neomycin > gentamicin
Max. ototoxic	Amikacin
Min ototoxic	Netilmicin
Min nm blockade	Tobramycin

Peripheral neuropathy:

- Stavudine
- Zalcitabine
- Ethambutol
- Oxaplatin
- Taxanes
- Metronidazole
- Didanosine
- INH
- Ethionamiide
- Alkylating agents
- Amiodarone
- Clofibrate

Receptor (ANS)	Site
Alpha 1	Blood vessels, dilator pupil, prostate, pilomotor, erection
Alpha 2	Presynaptic Platelet aggregation, decreases lipolysis, decreases insulin
Beta 1	Heart, JG cell increases rennin
Beta 2	Bronchus, GIT, bladder, liver, skeletal muscle, tremor, increases glucagon
M1	CNS, gastric glands, ganglion
M 2	Heart
M 3	Exocrine glands, smooth muscle, endothelium

Pseudocholinesterase

- Succinylcholine
- Ester local anesthetic
- Remifentanil
- Mivacurium
- Esmolol

Drugs used for urge incontinence

- Flavoxate
- Trospium
- Darifenacin
- Pantolamine
- Oxybutynin
- Tolferodine
- Solefenacin
- Tolazoline

BETA-BLOCKER PROPERTIES

Local anesthetic

- Propranolol
- Labetalol
- Pindolol
- Carvidilol
- Metoprolol
- Acebunolol
- Betoxolol

Lipid-insoluble

- Nadalol
- Atenolol
- Betoxolol
- Celiprolol
- Sotalol
- Acebutolol
- Bisoprolol

Intrinsic sympathomimetic activity

- Celiprolol
- Alprenolol
- Penbutolol
- Labetalol
- Pindalol
- Oxprenolol
- Acebutolol
- Carteolol

Isoprenaline	no alpha
Norepinephrine	no beta 2
Dobutamine	no D

Pharmacological sympathectomy—Guanethidine

Pharmacological defibrillator—Bretyllium

Floppy iris syndrome—Tamsulosin

Plasma Protein Binding

To albumin

- NSAID
- Phenytoin
- Warfarin
- Tolbutamide
- Valproic acid
- Benzodiazepine
- Sulfonamide

To alpha 2 glycoprotein

- Quinidine
- Morphine
- Propranolol
- Lidocaine
- Disopyramide

Least PBP

- Lithium
- Ethambutol
- Amikacin
- Ethosuccimide
- Acetaminophen
- Atenol

SIADH

- Nicotine
- TCA, MAO inhibitors
- Desmopressin
- Melphalan
- Clofibrate
- Thiazide
- Phenothiazine
- SSRI
- Oxytocin
- CBZ
- Clonidine
- Vinca alkaloids
- Treatment—water restriction, hypertonic saline, loop diuretic, demeclocycline, lithium, vaptans

Diabetes insipidus

- Demeclocycline
- Foscarnet
- Ethanol
- Propoxyphene
- Lithium
- Clozapine
- Amphotericin b
- Cisplatin

Treatment

Central

- Chlorpropamide
- Clofibrate
- CBZ
- Thiazide

Nephrogenic

- Amiloride
- Indomethacin
- Thiazide

G6PD HEMOLYSIS

Definite hemolysis

- Primaquine
- Sulfamethoxazole
- Nalidixic acid
- Naphtahalene
- Methylene blue
- Dapsone
- Clotrimazole
- Nitrofurantoin
- Niridazole
- Acetanilide

Possible hemolysis:

- Chloroquine
- Ciprofloxacin
- Aspirin
- Sulfasalazine
- Norfloxacin
- Vit k

Pyridoxine deficiency:

1. Cycloserine
2. Hydralazine
3. INH
4. Penicillamine

Dosage:

Lithium:

Prophylactic	0.5–0.8 meq/L
Therapeutic	0.8–1.2 meq/L
Toxic	> 1.5 meq/L

Magnesium sulfate:

Normal	< 3 meq/L
Therapeutic	4–7 meq/L
Absent knee jerk	> 10

THERAPEUTIC RANGES

Digoxin	0.8–2 ng/mL
Phenytoin	10–20 micrograms/mL
Theophylline	2–5 micrograms/mL
Lidocaine	5–20 micrograms/mL

Clinical trials

Preclinical	Animal testing	2.6 years
Phase I	Safety, kinetics	Clinical pharmacologist
Phase II	Efficacy > kinetics	Clinical pharm and clinical investigations
Phase III	Safety and efficacy	Clinical investigations
Postmarketing Phase IV	Adverse reactions	

Coronary steal phenomenon: Hydralazine, dipyridamole

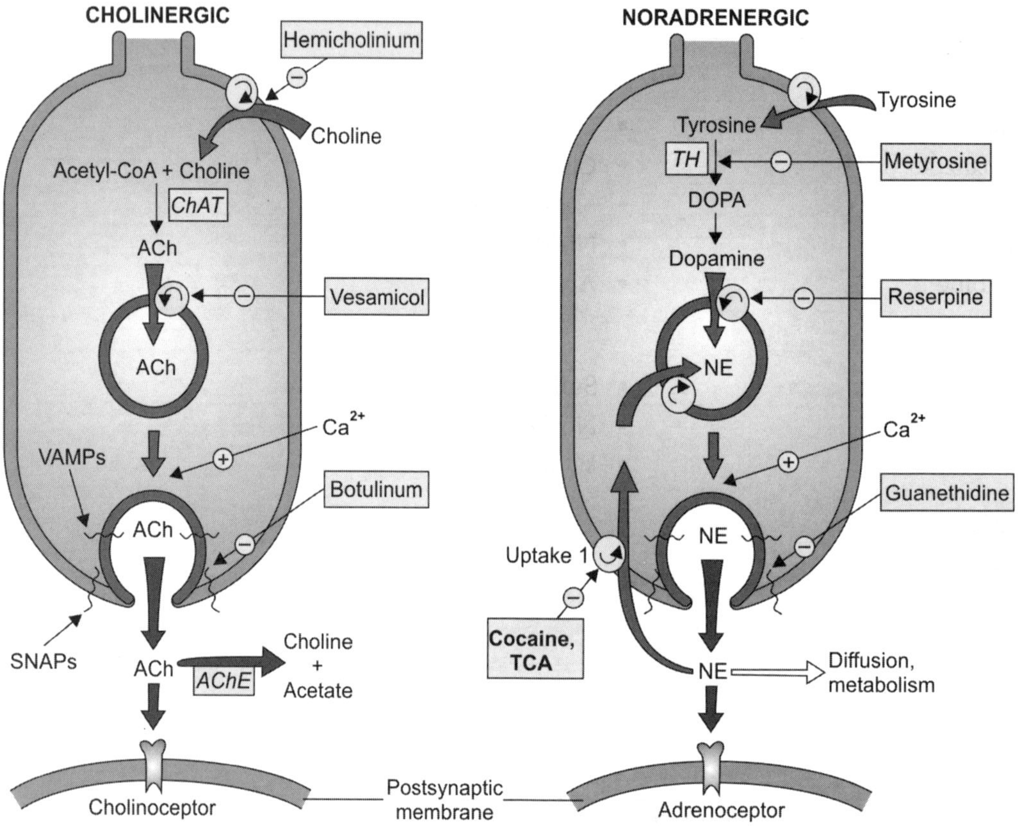

Fig. 4.1: Neuromuscular junction

AcetylCoA + Choline step inhibited by bromocetyl choline
Calcium channel inhibited by Aminoglycosides
dTC and Bungarotoxin (alpha: cobra, beta: krait) are direct AChR blockers
Black widow spider venom increases Ach release and subsequently causes paralysis
Carbechol: Maximum nicotinic activity, bethanechol has the least.

Prostaglandins

PGE1

Misoprostol: Peptic ulcer, cervical ripening
Rioprostol: NA in India
Alprostadol: Maintain PDA, erectile dysfunction

PGE 2

Dinoprostone: Second trimester MTP, cervical ripening
Enprostil: NA in India

PGF2-alpha

Dinoprost: Second trimester MTP
Carboprost: Second trimester MTP, PPH
Latanoprost: Glaucoma—increases UV outflow

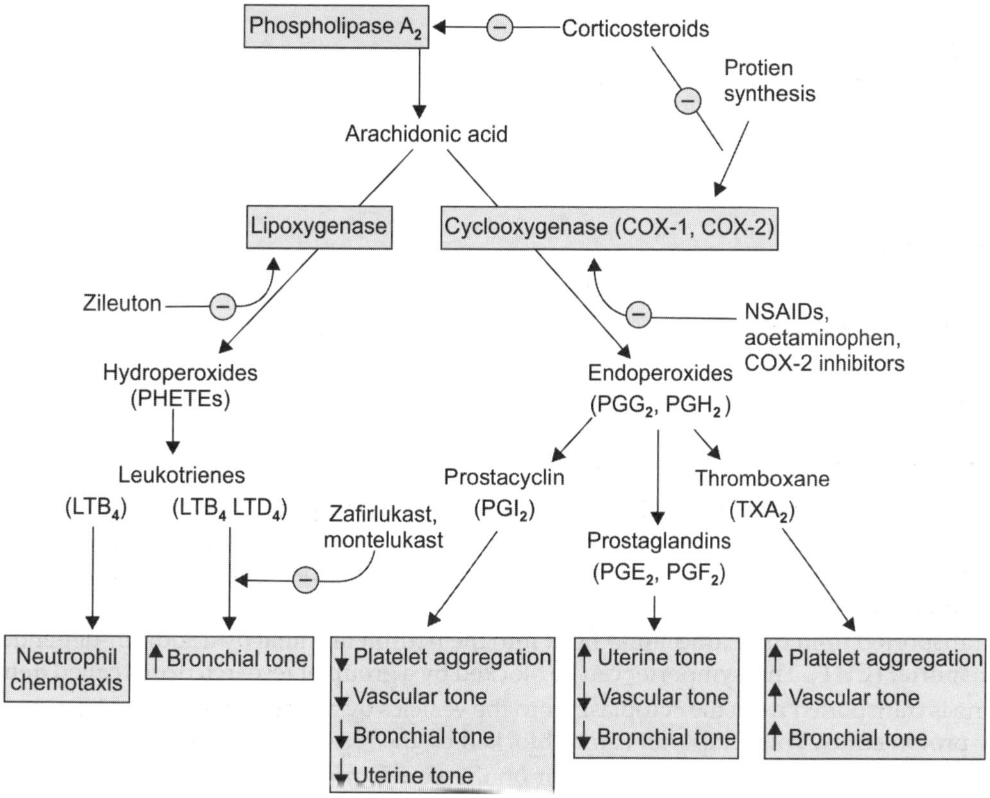

Steroids

Most potent glucocorticoids	Betamethasone
Least potent glucocorticoid	Cortisone
Maximum glucocorticoid activity	Dexamethasone
Most potent mineralocorticoid	Fludrocortisone
Maximum mineralocorticoid activity	Aldosterone
Zero mineralocorticoid activity—Methyl Pred, Triamcinolone, Dexa and Beta	
Zero glucocorticoid activity	DOCA
Glucocorticoid with maximum mineralocorticoid activity	Hydrocortisone

Drugs used for abstaining from smoking

- Mecamylamine
- Bupropion
- Varenicillin
- Amfebutamone

- Clonidine
- Topiramate
- Tryptophan
- Rimanobant
- Nortryptiline

Drugs in alcoholics

- Naltrexone (used in all substance disorders except smoking)
- Acamprosate
- BZD
- Ondansetron
- Disulfiram
- Topiramate
- Fluoxetine

Drugs used in heroin users

- Beta blockers
- Methadone
- Naltrexone
- Ioxfexidine
- Clonidine
- Buprenorphine
- Levomethadyl

Drugs for specific tumors

- HCC-sorafinib
- Kaposi-liposomal doxorubicin
- Pancreas-gemcitabine
- CLL-Fludarabine
- RCC-sunitinib
- Colon-FOLFOX regimen
- Hairy cell-cladribin

Autonomic Nervous System

- Vesicles are provided with **vesicle-associated membrane proteins (VAMPs),** which serve to align them with release sites on the inner neuronal cell membrane and participate in triggering the release of transmitter. The corresponding release site on the inner surface of the nerve terminal membrane contains **synaptosomal nerve-associated proteins (SNAPs).**
- Choline is transported from the extracellular fluid into the neuron terminal by a sodium-dependent membrane **choline transporter** (CHT). This symporter can be blocked by a group of research drugs called **hemicholiniums.**
- Acetylcholine is transported from the cytoplasm into the vesicles by a **vesicle-associated transporter (VAT)** that is driven by proton efflux. This antiporter can be blocked by the research drug **vesamicol.**
- Calcium interacts with the VAMP **synaptotagmin** on the vesicle membrane and triggers fusion of the vesicle membrane with the terminal membrane and opening of a pore into the synapse.
- The acetylcholine vesicle release process is blocked by **botulinum toxin** through the enzymatic removal of two amino acids from one or more of the fusion proteins.
- Another cholinesterase with a lower specificity for acetylcholine, butyrylcholinesterase [pseudocholinesterase], is found in blood plasma, liver, glia, and many other tissues.
- A few sympathetic fibers, such as those involved in sweating, are cholinergic.
- The conversion of tyrosine to dopa, is the rate-limiting step in catecholamine transmitter synthesis. It can be inhibited by the tyrosine analog **metyrosine.**
- A high-affinity antiporter for catecholamines located in the wall of the storage vesicle (**vesicular monoamine transporter, VMAT**) can be inhibited by the **reserpine** alkaloids. Reserpine causes depletion of transmitter stores.
- **Norepinephrine transporter, NET,** carries norepinephrine and similar molecules back into the cell cytoplasm from the synaptic cleft. NET is also commonly called uptake 1 or reuptake 1 and is partially responsible for the termination of synaptic activity. NET can be inhibited by **cocaine** and **tricyclic antidepressant** drugs, resulting in an increase of transmitter activity in the synaptic cleft.
- Release into cleft can be blocked by drugs such as guanethidine and bretylium.

- Indirectly acting and mixed sympathomimetics, e.g. **tyramine, amphetamines,** and **ephedrine,** are capable of releasing stored transmitter from noradrenergic nerve endings by a calcium-independent process.
- Capsaicin, a neurotoxin derived from chilli peppers, can cause the release of transmitter (especially substance P) from NANC (nonadrenergic noncholinergic) neurons and, if given in high doses, destruction of the neuron.
- The sensory fibers in the nonadrenergic, noncholinergic systems are probably better termed "sensory-efferent" or "sensory-local effector" fibers because, when activated by a sensory input, they are capable of releasing transmitter peptides from the sensory ending itself, from local axon branches, and from collaterals that terminate in the autonomic ganglia. These peptides are potent agonists in many autonomic effector tissues.
- Heart has M_2. Others (GIT, bronchi, eyes, etc.) have M_3. Endothelium secreting EDRF has M_5 in addition to M_3.
- Blood vessels have α_1. After that β_2 is most common. It relaxes. Heart has β_2 and β_1. Fat cells have β_3. Kidney has β_1.
- M_1, M_3, M_5 increase IP_3 and DAG. M_2, M_4 decreases cAMP and open up K^+ channels.
- β_2, β_1, β_3 all increases cAMP but are inhibitory. α_1 increases IP_3 and DAG. α_2 decreases cAMP.
- The *net* effect of ordinary pressor doses of norepinephrine in a normal subject is to produce a marked increase in peripheral vascular resistance, an increase in mean arterial pressure, and a consistent *slowing* of heart rate. Bradycardia, the reflex compensatory response elicited by this agent, is the *exact opposite* of the drug's direct action; yet it is completely predictable if the integration of cardiovascular function by the ANS is understood.
- Epinephrine and angiotensin have excitatory effects on adrenergic presynaptic neurons. Ach acting through Nm receptor on presynaptic neuron has autoexcitatory effect on presynaptic cholinergic neurons. Serotonin has an inhibitory effect on cholinergic preganglionic neurons.
- Ciliary muscle contraction causes accommodation of focus for near vision. Marked contraction of the ciliary muscle, which often occurs with cholinesterase inhibitor intoxication, is called *cyclospasm*.
- Acetyl choline, methacholine, carbachol, bethanechol.
- A state of "depolarizing blockade" occurs initially during persistent agonist occupancy of the receptor. Continued agonist occupancy is associated with return of membrane voltage to the resting level. The receptor becomes desensitized to agonist, and this state is refractory to reversal by other agonists.
- Intravenous infusions of minimally effective doses of acetylcholine in humans (e.g. 20–50 mcg/min) cause vasodilation, resulting in a reduction in blood pressure, often accompanied by a reflex increase in heart rate. Larger doses of acetylcholine produce bradycardia and decrease atrioventricular node conduction velocity in addition to hypotension.
- Parasympathetic innervation of the ventricles is much less extensive than that of the atria; activation of ventricular muscarinic receptors causes much less physiologic effect than that seen in atria. However, during sympathetic nerve stimulation, the effects of muscarinic agonists on ventricular function are clearly evident because of muscarinic modulation of sympathetic effects (accentuated antagonism).
- Pilocarpine acts on M_1 receptor.
- Pilocarpine is an interesting exception to the statement that cholinomimetics cause hypotension. If given intravenously (an experimental exercise), it may produce hypertension after a brief initial hypotensive response. The longer-lasting hypertensive effect can be traced to sympathetic ganglionic discharge caused by activation of postganglionic cell membrane M_1 receptors, which close K^+ channels and elicit slow excitatory (depolarizing) postsynaptic potentials. This effect, like the hypotensive effect, can be blocked by atropine, an antimuscarinic drug.
- The human uterus is not notably sensitive to muscarinic agonists.
- The M_1 subtype is richly expressed in brain areas involved in cognition. Knockout of M_1 receptors was associated with impaired neuronal plasticity in the forebrain, and pilocarpine did not induce seizures in M_1 mutant mice.
- Animals lacking M_3 receptors, especially those in the hypothalamus, had reduced appetite and diminished body fat mass.
- Acetylcholine regulates norepinephrine release via $\alpha3\beta4$ receptors in the hippocampus and inhibits acetylcholine release from neurons in the hippocampus and cortex. The $\alpha4\beta2$ oligomer, the most abundant nicotinic receptor in brain, has a high affinity for agonist.

- In high concentrations, nicotine induces tremor, emesis, and stimulation of the respiratory center. At still higher levels, nicotine causes convulsions, which may terminate in fatal coma. The lethal effects on the central nervous system and the fact that nicotine is readily absorbed form the basis for the use of nicotine as an insecticide.
- Edrophonium, neostigmine, and pyridostigmine are synthetic quaternary ammonium agents used in medicine.
- Physostigmine (eserine) is a naturally occurring tertiary amine of greater lipid solubility that is also used in therapeutics.
- Carbaryl (carbaril) is typical of a large group of carbamate insecticides designed for very high lipid solubility, so that absorption into the insect and distribution to its central nervous system are very rapid.
- Echothiophate, a thiocholine derivative, is of clinical value because it retains the very long duration of action of other organophosphates but is more stable in aqueous solution.
- Soman is an extremely potent "nerve gas."
- Parathion and malathion are thiophosphate (sulfur-containing phosphate) prodrugs that are inactive as such; they are converted to the phosphate derivatives in animals and plants and are used as insecticides.
- After the initial binding-hydrolysis step, the phosphorylated enzyme complex may undergo a process called **aging.** This process apparently involves the breaking of one of the oxygen-phosphorus bonds of the inhibitor and further strengthens the phosphorus-enzyme bond. The rate of aging varies with the particular organophosphate compound. For example, aging occurs within 10 minutes with the chemical warfare agent, soman, and in 48 hours with the agent, VX...
- If given before aging has occurred, strong nucleophiles like pralidoxime are able to break the phosphorus-enzyme bond and can be used as 'cholinesterase regenerator' drugs for organophosphate insecticide poisoning. Once aging has occurred, the enzyme-inhibitor complex is even more stable and is more difficult to break, even with oxime regenerator compounds.
- Three groups of cholinesterase inhibitors. 1. Alcohols (e.g. edrophonium) 2. Carbamates (e.g. physostigmine) 3. Organophosphates (e.g. echothiophates).
- Alcohols bind reversibly to the active site.
- Carbamates cause carbomylation.
- Organophosphates cause phosphorylation with aging phenomenon.
- First two are reversible. The third is not.
- Cholinesterase inhibitors: In the heart, the effects on the parasympathetic limb predominate. Thus, cholinesterase inhibitors such as edrophonium, physostigmine, or neostigmine mimic the effects of vagal nerve activation on the heart. Negative chronotropic, dromotropic, and inotropic effects are produced, and cardiac output falls.
- Cholinesterase inhibitors have minimal effects by direct action on vascular smooth muscle because most vascular beds lack cholinergic innervation (coronary vasculature is an exception).
- Some quaternary carbamate cholinesterase inhibitors, e.g. neostigmine, have an additional *direct* nicotinic agonist effect at the neuromuscular junction. This may contribute to the effectiveness of these agents as therapy for myasthenia.
- Accommodative esotropia (strabismus caused by hypermetropic accommodative error) in young children is sometimes diagnosed and treated with cholinomimetic agonists. Dosage is similar to or higher than that used for glaucoma.
- Of the choline esters, bethanechol is the most widely used for GI and UT disorders. Of the cholinesterase inhibitors, neostigmine is the most widely used for these applications.
- Pilocarpine has long been used to increase salivary secretion.
- Cevimeline, a quinuclidine derivative of acetylcholine, is a new direct-acting muscarinic agonist used for the treatment of dry mouth associated with Sjögren's syndrome and that caused by radiation damage of the salivary glands.
- Patients with myasthenia are exquisitely sensitive to the action of curariform drugs and other drugs that interfere with neuromuscular transmission, e.g. aminoglycoside antibiotics.
- Cholinesterase inhibitors—but not direct-acting acetylcholine receptor agonists—are extremely valuable as therapy for myasthenia. Patients with ocular myasthenia may be treated with cholinesterase inhibitors alone.

Patients having more widespread muscle weakness are also treated with immunosuppressant drugs (steroids, cyclosporine, and azathioprine).

- Long-term therapy for myasthenia gravis is usually accomplished with pyridostigmine; neostigmine or ambenonium are alternatives.
- The short-acting cholinesterase inhibitor edrophonium was used to treat supraventricular tachyarrhythmias, particularly paroxysmal supraventricular tachycardia. In this application, edrophonium has been replaced by newer drugs (adenosine and the calcium channel blockers verapamil and diltiazem).
- Tacrine is a drug with anticholinesterase and other cholinomimetic actions that has been used for the treatment of mild to moderate Alzheimer's disease. Tacrine's efficacy is modest, and hepatic toxicity is significant. Donepezil, galantamine, and rivastigmine are newer, more selective acetylcholinesterase inhibitors that appear to have the same modest clinical benefit as tacrine in treatment of cognitive dysfunction in Alzheimer's patients. Donepezil may be given once daily because of its long half-life and it lacks the hepatotoxic effect of tacrine. However, no trials comparing these newer drugs with tacrine have been reported.
- Nicotine replacement therapy, varenicline are effective help in cessation of smoking. Bupropion, an anti-depressant is also effective but lesser than varenicline.
- Chronic exposure to certain organophosphate compounds, including some organophosphate cholinesterase inhibitors, causes delayed neuropathy associated with demyelination of axons. **Triorthocresyl phosphate,** an additive in lubricating oils, is the prototype agent of this class. The effects are not caused by cholinesterase inhibition but rather by neuropathy target esterase (NTE) inhibition whose symptoms (weakness of upper and lower extremities, unsteady gait) appear 1–2 weeks after exposure.
- Cholinoreceptor blockers. Quaternary amines for GI applications. Propantheline and glycopyrrolate.
- Tertiary amines: Pirenzepine, dicyclomine, tropicamide.
- Quaternary amines used for asthma: Ipratropium, benztropine.
- M_1 receptor blockers: Pirenzepine, telenzepine, dicyclomine.
- M_2 receptor blockers: Gallamine, AF-DX 116.
- M_3 receptor blockers: Darifenacin, solifenacin, oxybutinin.
- Tissues most sensitive to atropine are the salivary, bronchial, and sweat glands. Secretion of acid by the gastric parietal cells is the least sensitive. In most tissues, antimuscarinic agents block exogenously administered cholinoceptor agonists more effectively than endogenously released acetylcholine.
- The sinoatrial node is very sensitive to muscarinic receptor blockade. Moderate to high therapeutic doses of atropine cause tachycardia in the innervated and spontaneously beating heart by blockade of vagal slowing. However, lower doses often result in initial bradycardia before the effects of peripheral vagal block become manifest. This slowing may be due to block of prejunctional M_1 receptors on vagal postganglionic fibers that normally limit acetylcholine release in the sinus node and other tissues.
- Antimuscarinic drugs are not as useful as the β-adrenoceptor stimulants in the treatment of asthma. The effectiveness of nonselective antimuscarinic drugs in treating chronic obstructive pulmonary disease (COPD) is limited because block of autoinhibitory M_2 receptors on postganglionic parasympathetic nerves can oppose the bronchodilation caused by block of M_3 receptors on airway smooth muscle.
- The antimuscarinic drugs have no significant effect on the uterus.
- Scopolamine is one of the oldest remedies for seasickness and is as effective as any more recently introduced agent.
- An ophthalmologic use of antimuscarinics (apart from its ability to cause mydriasis and cycloplegia) is to prevent synechia (adhesion) formation in uveitis and iritis. The longer-lasting preparations, especially homatropine, are valuable for this indication.
- **Ipratropium, a** synthetic analog of atropine, is used as an inhalational drug in asthma. Patients with COPD benefit from bronchodilators, especially antimuscarinic agents such as ipratropium and the recently approved **tiotropium.** In contrast to ipratropium, tiotropium has a longer bronchodilator action and can be given once daily. Tiotropium reduces the incidence of COPD exacerbations and is a useful adjunct to pulmonary rehabilitation in increasing exercise tolerance.

- Antimuscarinic agents can provide some relief in the treatment of common traveler's diarrhea and other mild or self-limited conditions of hypermotility. They are often combined with an opioid antidiarrheal drug, an extremely effective therapy. In this combination, however, the very low dosage of the antimuscarinic drug functions primarily to discourage abuse of the opioid agent. The classic combination of atropine with diphenoxylate, a nonanalgesic congener of meperidine, is available under many names (e.g. Lomotil) in both tablet and liquid form.
- **Oxybutynin,** which is somewhat selective for M_3 receptors, is used to relieve bladder spasm after urologic surgery, e.g. prostatectomy. It is also valuable in reducing involuntary voiding in patients with neurologic disease, e.g. children with meningomyelocele. **Trospium,** a nonselective antagonist, has been approved and is comparable in efficacy and side effects to oxybutynin.
- **Darifenacin** and **solifenacin** are recently approved antagonists that have greater selectivity for M_3 receptors than oxybutynin or trospium. Darifenacin and solifenacin have the advantage of once-daily dosing because of their long half-lives. **Tolterodine** and **fesoterodine,** M_3-selective antimuscarinics, are available for use in adults with urinary incontinence. They have many of the qualities of darifenacin and solifenacin and are available in extended-release tablets.
- Imipramine, a tricyclic antidepressant drug with strong antimuscarinic actions, has long been used to reduce incontinence in institutionalized elderly patients. It is moderately effective but causes significant CNS toxicity. Propiverine, a newer antimuscarinic agent, has been approved for this purpose.
- Large doses of atropine may be needed to oppose the muscarinic effects of extremely potent cholinesterase blocker agents like parathion and chemical warfare nerve gases: 1–2 mg of atropine sulfate may be given intravenously every 5–15 minutes until signs of effect (dry mouth, reversal of miosis) appear.
- A second class of compounds, capable of regenerating active enzyme from the organophosphorus-cholinesterase complex, is also available to treat organophosphorus poisoning. These oxime agents include pralidoxime (PAM), diacetylmonoxime (DAM), and others.
- At higher concentrations, atropine causes block of all parasympathetic functions. However, atropine is a remarkably safe drug *in adults*. Atropine poisoning has occurred as a result of attempted suicide, but most cases are due to attempts to induce hallucinations. Poisoned individuals manifest dry mouth, mydriasis, tachycardia, hot and flushed skin, agitation, and delirium for as long as 1 week. Body temperature is frequently elevated. These effects are memorialized in the adage, 'dry as a bone, blind as a bat, red as a beet, mad as a hatter.'
- Overdoses of atropine or its congeners are generally treated symptomatically. Symptomatic treatment may require temperature control with cooling blankets and seizure control with diazepam.
- Nicotinic ganglionic blockers: Hexamethonium, tetraethyl ammonium (TEA)
- Decamethonium is a depolarizing neuromuscular blocker.
- **Mecamylamine,** a secondary amine, was developed to improve the degree and extent of absorption from the gastrointestinal tract because the quaternary amine ganglion-blocking compounds were poorly and erratically absorbed after oral administration. **Trimethaphan,** a short-acting ganglion blocker, is inactive orally and is given by intravenous infusion.
- Hexamethonium actually produces most of its blockade by occupying sites in or on the nicotinic ion channel, not by occupying the cholinoceptor itself. In contrast, trimethaphan appears to block the nicotinic receptor, not the channel pore. Blockade can be surmounted by increasing the concentration of an agonist, e.g. acetylcholine.
- Mecamylamine blocks central nicotinic receptors and has been advocated as a possible adjunct with the transdermal nicotine patch to reduce nicotine craving in patients attempting to quit smoking.
- Trimethaphan is occasionally used in the treatment of hypertensive emergencies and dissecting aortic aneurysm; in producing hypotension, which can be of value in neurosurgery to reduce bleeding in the operative field; and in the treatment of patients undergoing electroconvulsive therapy. The toxicity of the ganglion-blocking drugs is limited to the autonomic effects already described. For most patients, these effects are intolerable except for acute use.
- Adrenoreceptors were initially characterized pharmacologically, with α-receptors having the comparative potencies epinephrine ≥ norepinephrine >> isoproterenol, and β-receptors having the comparative potencies isoproterenol > epinephrine ≥ norepinephrine.

- Indeed, some of the effects of α_2 adrenoceptors are independent of their ability to inhibit adenylyl cyclase; for example, α_2-receptor agonists cause platelet aggregation and a decrease in platelet cAMP levels, but it is not clear whether aggregation is the result of the decrease in cAMP or other mechanisms involving G_i-regulated effectors.
- The D_1 receptor is typically associated with the stimulation of adenylyl cyclase (Table 9–1); for example, D_1-receptor-induced smooth muscle relaxation is presumably due to cAMP accumulation in the smooth muscle of those vascular beds in which dopamine is a vasodilator. D_2 receptors have been found to inhibit adenylyl cyclase activity, open potassium channels, and decrease calcium influx.
- Phenylephrine, methoxamine α_1 selective.
- Clonidine, methylnorepinephrine α_2 selective.
- Dobutamine is β_1 selective.
- Albuterol, terbutaline, metaproterenol, ritodrine are β_2 selective.
- Fenoldopam is D_1 specific.
- A major mechanism of desensitization that occurs rapidly involves phosphorylation of receptors by members of the **G protein-coupled receptor kinase (GRK)** family, of which there are seven members. Phosphorylation of these receptors enhances their affinity for β-**arrestins**, a family of four widely expressed proteins. Upon binding of a β-arrestin molecule, the capacity of the receptor to activate G proteins is blunted, presumably as a result of steric hindrance. Arrestin then interacts with clathrin and clathrin adaptor AP2, leading to endocytosis of the receptor.
- Often, distinct polymorphisms occur in specific combination termed **haplotypes**. Some of these polymorphisms have been consistently shown to alter the susceptibility to diseases such as heart failure, to alter the propensity of a receptor to desensitize, and to alter therapeutic responses to drugs in diseases such as asthma.
- Increasing the size of alkyl substituents on the amino group tends to increase β-receptor activity.
- α_2 receptor activation causes platelet aggregation and inhibition of lipolysis.
- Effect of epinephrine on total peripheral resistance: Small doses decrease. Large doses increase. But venous tone always increases.
- Effect of phenylephrine on heart rate. It acts on the α_1 receptor selectively. So it increases the total peripheral vascular resistance. This causes a reflex decrease in the heart rate.
- The α-agonist midodrine is commonly used to ameliorate orthostatic hypotension in patients with pure autonomic failure or with diabetic neuropathy.
- α2-agonists are used as sympatholytics in the treatment of hypertension.
- In smooth muscles if you increase the cAMP it relaxes (β receptor stimulation decreases the peripheral resistance). But if you decrease the cAMP it contracts (as evident by the α_2 receptor stimulation which decreases the cAMP concentration)
- Physiologic stimulation of the heart by catecholamines tends to increase coronary blood flow.
- Intravenous administration of dopamine promotes vasodilation of renal, splanchnic, coronary, cerebral, and perhaps other resistance vessels, via activation of D_1 receptors.
- Beta-receptor activation promotes the relaxation of smooth muscle by increasing the cAMP! Although the mechanism of the smooth muscle effect is uncertain, it may involve the phosphorylation of myosin light-chain kinase to an inactive form.
- Dopamine at low doses: peripheral resistance may decrease. At higher rates of infusion, dopamine activates vascular α-receptors, leading to vasoconstriction, including in the renal vascular bed. Consequently, high rates of infusion of dopamine may mimic the actions of epinephrine.
- Activation of β_2 adrenoceptors by endogenous epinephrine or by sympathomimetic drugs promotes the uptake of potassium into cells, leading to a fall in extracellular potassium. This may lead to a fall in the plasma potassium concentration during stress or protect against a rise in plasma potassium during exercise.
- Renin secretion is stimulated by β_1 and inhibited by α_2 receptors; indeed, β-receptor antagonist drugs may lower blood pressure in patients with hypertension at least in part by lowering plasma renin.
- **Midodrine** is a prodrug that is enzymatically hydrolyzed to desglymidodrine, a selective α_1-receptor agonist.

- **α_2-selective agonists** have an important ability to decrease blood pressure through actions in the central nervous system even though direct application to a blood vessel may cause vasoconstriction. Such drugs (e.g. **clonidine, methyldopa, guanfacine, guanabenz**) are useful in the treatment of hypertension. **Dexmedetomidine** is a centrally acting α_2-selective agonist that is indicated for sedation of initially intubated and mechanically ventilated patients during treatment in an intensive care setting. It also reduces the requirements for opioids in pain control.
- **Xylometazoline** and **oxymetazoline** are direct-acting α agonists. These drugs have been used as topical decongestants because of their ability to promote constriction of the nasal mucosa. When taken in large doses, oxymetazoline may cause hypotension, presumably because of a central clonidine-like effect (see Chapter 11). Oxymetazoline has significant affinity for α_{2A} receptors.
- Beta$_1$-selective agents include **dobutamine** and a partial agonist, **prenalterol**
- **Methamphetamine** (*N*-methylamphetamine) is very similar to amphetamine with an even higher ratio of central to peripheral actions. **Phenmetrazine** is a variant phenylisopropylamine with amphetamine-like effects. It has been promoted as an anorexiant and is also a popular drug of abuse. **Methylphenidate** is an amphetamine variant whose major pharmacologic effects and abuse potential are similar to those of amphetamine. Methylphenidate may be effective in some children with attention deficit hyperactivity disorder. **Modafinil** is a psychostimulant that differs from amphetamine in structure, neurochemical profile, and behavioral effects. Its mechanism of action is not fully known; it inhibits both norepinephrine and dopamine transporters and it increases interstitial concentrations not only of norepinephrine and dopamine, but also serotonin and glutamate while decreasing GABA levels. It is used primarily to improve wakefulness in narcolepsy and some other conditions.
- **Atomoxetine** is a selective inhibitor of the norepinephrine reuptake transporter. Its actions, therefore, are mediated by potentiation of norepinephrine levels in noradrenergic synapses. It is used in the treatment of attention deficit disorders. Atomoxetine has surprisingly little cardiovascular effect because it has a clonidine-like effect in the central nervous system to decrease sympathetic outflow while at the same time potentiating the effects of norepinephrine in the periphery.
- **Sibutramine** is a serotonin and norepinephrine reuptake inhibitor and is the only appetite suppressant approved by the FDA for long-term treatment of obesity.
- **Duloxetine** is also a widely used antidepressant with serotonin and norepinephrine reuptake inhibitory effects.
- Long-acting topical decongestants include xylometazoline and oxymetazoline. Most of these mucous membrane decongestants are available as over-the-counter products.
- Dipivefrin is the prodrug of epinephrine.
- **Apraclonidine** and **brimonidine** are α_2-selective agonists that also lower intraocular pressure and are approved for use in glaucoma. The mechanism of action of these drugs in treating glaucoma is still uncertain; direct neuroprotective effects may be involved in addition to the benefits of lowering intraocular pressure.
- **Ritodrine, terbutaline,** and similar drugs have been used to suppress premature labor.
- **Modafinil,** a new amphetamine substitute, is approved for use in narcolepsy and is claimed to have fewer disadvantages (excessive mood changes, insomnia and abuse potential) than amphetamine in this condition. The appetite-suppressing effect of these agents is easily demonstrated in experimental animals.
- Phentolamine and prazosin are examples of reversible antagonists.
- Phenoxybenzamine, an agent related to the nitrogen mustards, forms a reactive ethyleneimonium intermediate that covalently binds to α-receptors, resulting in irreversible blockade.
- Alpha-receptor antagonists often cause orthostatic hypotension and reflex tachycardia; nonselective ($\alpha_1 = \alpha_2$) blockers usually cause significant tachycardia if blood pressure is lowered below normal. Orthostatic hypotension is due to antagonism of sympathetic nervous system stimulation of α_1 receptors in vascular smooth muscle; contraction of veins is an important component of the normal capacity to maintain blood pressure in the upright position since it decreases venous pooling in the periphery. Constriction of arterioles in the legs also contributes to the normal orthostatic response. Tachycardia may be more marked with agents that block α_2-presynaptic receptors in the heart, since the augmented release of norepinephrine will further stimulate β-receptors in the heart.
- Prazosin, terazosin, doxazosin are $\alpha_1$selective antagonists.

- Phentolamine is nonselective α blocker.
- Yohimbine, tolazoline are α_2 selective blockers.
- Labetalol and carvedilol are mixed antagonists with both α and β actions.
- Butoxamine is β_2 selective blocker.
- Most adverse effects of phenoxybenzamine derive from its α-receptor-blocking action; the most important are orthostatic hypotension and tachycardia. Nasal stuffiness and inhibition of ejaculation also occur. Since phenoxybenzamine enters the central nervous system, it may cause less specific effects, including fatigue, sedation, and nausea. Because phenoxybenzamine is an alkylating agent, it may have other adverse effects that have not yet been characterized.
- Phentolamine also has minor inhibitory effects at serotonin receptors and agonist effects at muscarinic and H_1 and H_2 histamine receptors.
- **Alfuzosin** is an α_1-selective quinazoline derivative that is approved for use in BPH (benign prostatic hyperplasia)
- **Urapidil** is an α_1 antagonist (its primary effect) that also has weak α_2-agonist and 5-HT_{1A}-agonist actions and weak antagonist action at β_1 receptors. It is used in Europe as an antihypertensive agent and for benign prostatic hyperplasia.
- It is interesting that the use of α-adrenoceptor antagonists such as prazosin has been found to be associated with either no changes in plasma lipids or increased concentrations of high-density lipoproteins (HDL), which could be a favorable alteration. The mechanism for this effect is not known.
- Betaxolol, penbutolol, pindolol, and sotalol have low first-pass metabolism and hence they have a high bioavailability.
- Esmolol is rapidly hydrolyzed and has a half-life of approximately 10 minutes.
- The cytochrome P450 2D6 (CYP2D6) genotype is a major determinant of interindividual differences in metoprolol plasma clearance.
- Nadolol is excreted unchanged in the urine and has the longest half-life of any available β antagonist (up to 24 hours). The half-life of nadolol is prolonged in renal failure.
- Sotalol is a nonselective β-receptor antagonist that lacks local anesthetic action but has marked class III antiarrhythmic effects, reflecting potassium channel blockade.
- **Nebivolol** is the most highly selective β_1-adrenergic receptor blocker, and it has the additional quality of eliciting vasodilation. This may be due to a poorly understood stimulation of the endothelial nitric oxide pathway.
- **Timolol** is a nonselective agent with no local anesthetic activity. It has excellent ocular hypotensive effects when administered topically in the eye.
- **Pindolol, acebutolol, carteolol, bopindolol,** * **oxprenolol,** * **celiprolol,** * and **penbutolol** are of interest because they have partial β-agonist activity.
- Celiprolol is a β_1-selective antagonist with a modest capacity to activate β_2 receptors.
- Carvedilol also appears to attenuate oxygen free radical-initiated lipid peroxidation and to inhibit vascular smooth muscle mitogenesis independently of adrenoceptor blockade. These effects may contribute to the clinical benefits of the drug in chronic heart failure
- **Butoxamine** is a research drug selective for β_2 receptors. Selective β_2-blocking drugs have not been actively sought because there is no obvious clinical application for them; none is available for clinical use.
- Sotalol has antiarrhythmic effects involving ion channel blockade in addition to its β-blocking action.
- Systemic administration of β-blocking drugs for other indications was found serendipitously to reduce intraocular pressure in patients with glaucoma. Subsequently, it was found that topical administration also reduces intraocular pressure. The mechanism appears to involve reduced production of aqueous humor by the ciliary body, which is physiologically activated by cAMP.
- A life-threatening adverse cardiac effect of a β antagonist may be overcome directly with isoproterenol or with glucagon (glucagon stimulates the heart via glucagon receptors, which are not blocked by β antagonists), but neither of these methods is without hazard.
- Some anesthetics, such as halothane, may sensitize the heart to the arrhythmogenic effects of sympathomimetic agents.

- HE COMB—Antihistaminics, antiemetics, anticholinergics, opioids, skeletal muscle relaxants, barbiturates and benzodiazepines are adjuvants to anesthesia.
- There has been at least one report that transient use of nitrous oxide can cause aplastic anemia in the unborn child. Oral clefts have occurred in the fetuses of women who have received benzodiazepines. Diazepam should not be used routinely during labor, because it results in temporary hypotonia and altered thermoregulation in the newborn.
- For children, without intravenous access, nonpungent agents, such as halothane or sevoflurane, are used to induce general anesthesia. This is termed inhalation induction.
- The solubility in blood is ranked in the following order: halothane > enflurane > isoflurane > sevoflurane > desflurane > nitrous oxide. (Heavy elegant iguanas strangle distant nations)
- Neurogenic pain responds best to anticonvulsants (for example pregabalin), tricyclic antidepressants (for example, amitriptyline), or serotonin/norepinephrine reuptake inhibitors (for example, duloxetine) rather than NSAIDs or opioids.
- Morphine produces a powerful sense of contentment and well-being. Euphoria may be caused by disinhibition of the ventral tegmentum.
- The pinpoint pupil, characteristic of morphine use, results from stimulation of μ and κ receptors. Morphine excites the Edinger-Westphal nucleus of the oculomotor nerve, which causes enhanced parasympathetic stimulation to the eye.
- Morphine may prolong the second stage of labor by transiently decreasing the strength, duration, and frequency of uterine contractions.
- Morphine suppresses the cough reflex; however, codeine or dextromethorphan are more widely used for this purpose. Codeine has greater antitussive action than morphine.
- Intravenous (IV) morphine dramatically relieves dyspnea caused by pulmonary edema associated with left ventricular failure possibly by its vasodilatory effect.
- Only a small percentage of morphine crosses the blood-brain barrier, because morphine is the least lipophilic of the common opioids. This contrasts with the more fat-soluble opioids, such as fentanyl, methadone, and heroin, which readily penetrate into the brain.
- Repeated use produces tolerance to the respiratory depressant, analgesic, euphoric, and sedative effects of morphine. However, tolerance usually does not develop to the pupil-constricting and constipating effects of the drug.
- Meperidine provides analgesia for any type of severe pain. Unlike morphine, meperidine is not clinically useful in the treatment of diarrhea or cough. Meperidine produces less of an increase in urinary retention than does morphine. (Despite being an antimuscarinic). It has significantly less effects on uterine smooth muscle than morphine and is the opioid commonly employed in obstetrics.
- Large or repetitive doses of meperidine can cause anxiety, tremors, muscle twitches, and rarely, convulsions due to the accumulation of a toxic metabolite, normeperidine.
- Fentanyl is often used during cardiac surgery because of its negligible effects on myocardial contractility.
- Sufentanil is even more potent than fentanyl.
- Heroin does not occur naturally. It is produced by diacetylation of morphine, which leads to a three-fold increase in its potency. Its greater lipid solubility allows it to cross the blood-brain barrier more rapidly than morphine, causing a more exaggerated euphoria when the drug is taken by injection.
- Propoxyphene is a derivative of methadone.
- Respiratory depression and sedation of propoxyphene can be antagonized by naloxone, but the cardiotoxicity cannot.
- A major use of buprenorphine is in opiate detoxification like methadone.
- Nalbuphine and butorphanol have a propensity to cause psychotomimetic (actions mimics the symptoms of psychosis) effects, but it is less than that of pentazocine.
- Nalbuphine does not affect the heart or increase blood pressure.
- Naltrexone is hepatotoxic.

- Nalmefene is a parenteral opioid antagonist.
- Drugs that are effective in seizure reduction accomplish this by a variety of mechanisms, including blockade of voltage-gated channels (Na^+ or Ca^{2+}), enhancement of inhibitory GABAergic impulses, or interference with excitatory glutamate transmission.
- Proposed mechanisms of action of Divalproex sodium include sodium channel blockade, blockade of GABA transaminase, and action at the T-type calcium channels.
- Fluoxetine is metabolized to an active product, norfluoxetine, which may have plasma concentrations greater than those of fluoxetine. The elimination half-life of norfluoxetine is about three times longer than fluoxetine and contributes to the longest half-life of all the SSRIs. As a result, fluoxetine has to be discontinued 4 weeks or longer before an MAOI can be administered to mitigate the risk of serotonin syndrome.
- Fluoxetine and paroxetine are potent inhibitors of the CYP2D6 isoenzyme, in contrast, fluvoxamine is an inhibitor of CYP3A4.
- The TCAs are substrates of the CYP2D6 system, and the serum levels of these agents tend to be substantially influenced by concurrent administration of drugs such as fluoxetine. In addition, genetic polymorphism for CYP2D6 may result in low or extensive metabolism of the TCAs.
- Trazodone and nefazodone are serotonin receptor blockers.
- Trazodone is mainly used as a sedative and not as an antidepressant.
- Nefazodone is a potent inhibitor of the CYP3A4 system and may interact with drugs metabolized by this enzyme.
- TCAs such as doxepin are sometimes prescribed as hypnotics and used in treatments for pruritus because of their antihistamine properties.
- Bupropion has virtually no direct effects on the serotonin system. It increases norepinephrine and dopamine.
- Mirtazapine has a complex pharmacology. It is an antagonist of the presynaptic α_2 autoreceptor and enhances the release of both norepinephrine and 5-HT. In addition, mirtazapine is an antagonist of 5-HT_2 and 5-HT_3 receptors. Finally, mirtazapine is a potent H_1 antagonist, which is associated with the drug's sedative effects.
- Unlike the TCAs or other antidepressants, amoxapine is a moderate inhibitor of the postsynaptic D_2 receptor. As such, amoxapine possesses some antipsychotic properties.
- Phenelzine and tranylcypromine are examples of irreversible, nonselective MAOIs.
- Several SSRIs and venlafaxine are approved for the treatment of social anxiety.
- The SNRI duloxetine was the first antidepressant to secure FDA approval for the treatment of pain associated with diabetic neuropathy and fibromyalgia.
- The SSRIs are known to be beneficial to many women with PMDD, and fluoxetine and sertraline have been approved for this indication.
- The SNRI duloxetine is approved in Europe for the treatment of urinary stress incontinence.
- Clopiramine and fluvoxamine and other SSRI's in OCD. So it is serotonin that helps.
- Trazodone priapism
- Nefazodone hepatotoxicity
- Amoxapine is sometimes associated with a parkinsonian syndrome due to its D_2-blocking action.
- Nefazodone is an inhibitor of the CYP3A4 isoenzyme, so it can raise the level and thus exacerbate adverse effects of many 3A4-dependent drugs. For example, triazolam levels are increased by concurrent administration of nefazodone such that a reduction in triazolam dosage by 75% is recommended.
- The serotonin syndrome is thought to be caused by overstimulation of 5-HT receptors in the central gray nuclei and the medulla. Symptoms range from mild to lethal and include a triad of cognitive (delirium, coma), autonomic (hypertension, tachycardia, diaphoreses) and somatic (myoclonus, hyperreflexia, tremor) effects.
- Some opioids, e.g. nalbuphine, are capable of producing an agonist (or partial agonist) effect at one opioid receptor subtype and an antagonist effect at another.
- Calcium blockers (ziconotide) can block pain transmission by inhibiting presynaptic release of glumate. This pain transmission can also be blocked by drugs that increase synaptic concentrations of norepinephrine by blocking reuptake (tapentadol).

- Butorphanol and nalbuphine have shown some clinical success as analgesics, but they can cause dysphoric reactions and have limited potency. It is interesting that butorphanol has also been shown to cause significantly greater analgesia in women than in men. In fact, gender-based differences in analgesia mediated by μ and δ-receptor activation have been widely reported.
- **Capsaicin receptor, TRPV1, TRPA1, P2X, Nav1.8, are the receptors for pain.**
- **Lidocaine** and **mexiletine**, which are useful in some chronic pain states, may act by blocking Nav1.8 (voltage gated sodium channel).
- **Ziconotide,** a blocker of voltage-gated N-type calcium channels, is approved for intrathecal analgesia in patients with refractory chronic pain. It is a synthetic peptide related to the marine snail toxin ω-conotoxin, which selectively blocks these calcium channels.
- In addition to the development of tolerance, persistent administration of opioid analgesics has been observed to *increase* the sensation of pain leading to a state of hyperalgesia. This phenomenon has been observed with several opioid analgesics, including morphine, fentanyl, and remifentanil. Spinal dynorphin and activation of the bradykinin receptor have emerged as important candidates for the mediation of opioid-induced hyperalgesia.
- Marked sedation occurs more frequently with compounds closely related to the phenanthrene derivatives (like morphine) and less frequently with the synthetic agents such as meperidine and fentanyl.
- Codeine in particular has been used to advantage in persons suffering from pathologic cough and in patients in whom it is necessary to maintain ventilation via an endotracheal tube. However, cough suppression by opioids may allow accumulation of secretions and thus lead to airway obstruction and atelectasis.
- Administration of μ-opioid receptor agonists such as morphine administered to the anterior hypothalamus produces hyperthermia, whereas administration of κ-agonists induces hypothermia.
- The opioids contract biliary smooth muscle, which can result in biliary colic. The sphincter of oddi may constrict, resulting in reflux of biliary and pancreatic secretions and elevated plasma amylase and lipase levels.
- μ opioids have been found to have an antidiuretic effect in humans. Mechanisms may involve both the CNS and peripheral sites. Opioids also enhance renal tubular sodium reabsorption.
- Occasionally, ureteral colic caused by a renal calculus is made worse by opioid-induced increase in ureteral tone.
- Buprenorphine is an opioid agonist that displays high binding affinity but low intrinsic activity at the μ receptor. Its slow rate of dissociation from the μ receptor has also made it an attractive alternative to methadone for the management of opioid withdrawal. Pentazocine and nalbuphine are other examples of opioid analgesics with mixed agonist-antagonist properties. It is BPN. Below Poverty Na?
- In addition, stimulant drugs such as the amphetamines have been shown to enhance the analgesic actions of the opioids and thus may be very useful adjuncts in the patient with chronic pain.
- The phenylpiperidine drugs (e.g. meperidine) appear to produce less depression, particularly respiratory depression, in newborn infants than does morphine; this may justify their use in obstetric practice.
- The relief produced by intravenous morphine in dyspnea from pulmonary edema associated with left ventricular heart failure is remarkable.
- Synthetic surrogates with more selective gastrointestinal effects and few or no CNS effects, e.g. diphenoxylate or loperamide, are used.
- Butorphanol is the only opioid currently available in the USA in a nasal formulation, but more are expected.
- NMDA-receptor antagonists (e.g. ketamine) have shown promise in preventing or reversing opioid-induced tolerance in animals and humans
- The signs and symptoms of withdrawal from an opioid agonist include rhinorrhea, lacrimation, yawning, chills, gooseflesh (piloerection), hyperventilation, hyperthermia, mydriasis, muscular aches, vomiting, diarrhea, anxiety, and hostility.
- In addition to methadone, buprenorphine and clonidine (an α_2-noradrenergic receptor agonist) are FDA-approved treatments for opioid analgesic detoxification.
- Combining full agonist with partial agonist opioids should be avoided.
- Patients with adrenal insufficiency (Addison's disease) and those with hypothyroidism (myxedema) may have prolonged and exaggerated responses to opioids.

- **Interaction with Opioids:** Monoamine oxidase inhibitors: Relative contraindication to all opioid analgesics because of the high incidence of hyperpyrexic coma; hypertension has also been reported.
- **Morphine, hydromorphone,** and **oxymorphone** are strong agonists useful in treating severe pain. These prototypic agents have been described in detail above.
- Methadone is widely used in the treatment of opioid abuse.
- For detoxification of a heroin-dependent addict, low doses of methadone (5–10 mg orally) are given two or three times daily for 2 or 3 days. Upon discontinuing methadone, the addict experiences a mild but endurable withdrawal syndrome.
- F SAR Fentanyl, Sufentanyl, Alfentanyl, Remifentanyl.
- Sufentanil is five to seven times more potent than fentanyl. Alfentanil is considerably less potent than fentanyl, but acts more rapidly and has a markedly shorter duration of action. Remifentanil is metabolized very rapidly by blood and nonspecific tissue esterases, making its pharmacokinetic and pharmacodynamic half-lives extremely short.
- **Levorphanol** is a synthetic opioid analgesic closely resembling morphine in its action.
- **Codeine, dihydrocodeine, oxycodone** and **hydrocodone** are all somewhat less efficacious than morphine (they are partial agonists)
- **Diphenoxylate** and its metabolite, **difenoxin,** are not used for analgesia but for the treatment of diarrhea. **Loperamide** is a phenylpiperidine derivative used to control diarrhea.
- Moreover, buprenorphine is also available combined with a pure μ-opioid antagonist (Suboxone) to help prevent its diversion for illicit intravenous abuse.
- Nalbuphine has a ceiling effect when it comes to respiratory depression. However respiratory depression that does occur is irreversible by naloxone.
- **Butorphanol** produces analgesia equivalent to nalbuphine and buprenorphine but appears to produce more sedation at equianalgesic doses. Butorphanol is considered to be predominantly a κ-agonist. However, it may also act as a partial agonist or antagonist at the μ-receptor.
- The opioid derivatives most commonly used as antitussives are dextromethorphan, codeine, levopropoxyphene, and noscapine (DC looks nice where DC is the custom car designer).
- The pure opioid antagonist drugs are **naloxone, naltrexone** and **nalmefene**.
- Careful titration of the naloxone dosage can often eliminate the itching, nausea, and vomiting while sparing the analgesia. For this purpose, oral naloxone, and more recently modified analogs of naloxone and naltrexone, have been approved by the FDA. These include **methylnaltrexone bromide** (Relistor) for the treatment of constipation in patients with late-stage advanced illness and **alvimopan** (Entereg) for the treatment of postoperative ileus following bowel resection surgery.
- Levodopa should not be given to psychotic patients because it may exacerbate the mental disturbance. It is also contraindicated in patients with angle-closure glaucoma. Careful in arrhythmia, and peptic ulcer and history of melanoma.
- Apomorphine is a potent dopamine agonist but is discussed separately in a later section in this chapter because it is used primarily as a rescue drug for patients with disabling response fluctuations to levodopa.
- Bromocriptine is excreted in the bile and feces.
- Pergolide, another ergot derivative, directly stimulates both D_1 and D_2 receptors. The drug is no longer available because its use has been associated with the development of valvular heart disease.
- The dopamine agonist rotigotine, delivered daily through a skin patch, was approved in 2007 by the FDA for treatment of early Parkinson's disease. The product was recalled in 2008 because of crystal formation on the patches, affecting the availability and efficacy of the agonist.
- Confusion, hallucinations, delusions, and other psychiatric reactions are potential complications of dopaminergic treatment and are more common and severe with dopamine receptor agonists than with levodopa.
- Tolcapone is associated with hepatotoxicity. However, tolcapone has both central and peripheral effects, whereas the effect of entacapone is peripheral. The half-life of both drugs is approximately 2 hours, but tolcapone is slightly more potent and has a longer duration of action.

- Reserpine and the related drug tetrabenazine deplete biogenic monoamines from their storage sites, whereas haloperidol, metoclopramide, and the phenothiazines block dopamine receptors.
- **Rabbit syndrome,** another neuroleptic-induced disorder, is manifested by rhythmic vertical movements about the mouth; it may respond to anticholinergic drugs.
- **Coronary steal phenomenon:**
  - Hydralazine
  - Dipyridamole
- **Digoxin Excretion decreased by (hence level increased)**
  Antiarrhythmic agents
  - Quinidine — Class 1A; combined sodium and potassium channel blockade, intermediate kinetics
  - Propafenone — Class 1C; Sodium channel blockade, slow kinetics
  - Amiodarone — Class 3; potassium channel blockade
  - Verapamil — Class 4; Calcium channel blockers
  - Diltiazem — Class 4; Calcium channel blockers
  - → All these drugs blocks: P-glycoprotein
- **Digoxin *Level* decreased by**
  - Metoclopramide
  - Kaolin
  - Cholestyramine
  - Sulfasalazine
- **Digoxin *contraindicated* in:**
  - **Wolff–Parkinson–White syndrome (WPW)**
  - **Hypertrophic Obstructive Cardiomyopathy (HOCM)**

Why

- **Niacin – decreases hormone sensitive lipase (PPARα)**
- **Fibrate – Increases Lipoprotein lipase**
- **Hydralazine + IsoSorbide DiNitrate (ISDN) = Synergistic (decreases free radicals)**
  - *Guanethidine*, *Reserpine*, *Bretylium* → **Adrenergic neuron blockade**
  - Sodium nitroprusside, ACEs and ARBs, Hydralazine → Acts on **both artery and vein**
  - Hydralazine, Diazoxide, Calcium channel blockers → Acts mainly on **artery**
- **Fenoldopam: A selective D1 receptor partial agonist**
- Prolonged/high-dose intravenous (IV) therapy of sodium nitroprusside causes *Cyanide toxicity* with psychosis, weakness, hypothyroidism.
- **Subarachnoid Hemorrhage (SAH): Nimodipine is useful to reduce intracranial vasospasm.**
  - Captopril, Lisinopril → **Active drug** (all other ACEIs are prodrugs)
  - Simvastatin, Lovastatin → **Prodrug**

- Fosinopril
- Moexipril

→ [remember as **FM—no renal**]

except renal?

- Flecainide—Wolff–Parkinson–White syndrome (WPW)
- Ibutilide—Atrial Fibrillation (AF)
- Pravastatin – Confined to liver
- No myopathy
- Metabolized in the small intestine by sulfation
- Nonmicrosomal metabolization
- **Torsade de pointes (TdP)**
  - Treatment: **Isoproterenol**
  - Magnesium sulfate ($MgSO_4$)
  - Class 1b antiarrhythmic agents (decrease ADP)
  - Adriamycin = Doxorubicin
  - Rubidomycin = Daunorubicin
  - Plicamycin = Mithramycin
- **Purines:**
  - 6-Mercaptopurine [6-MP]
  - 6-Thioguanine [6-TG]
  - Fludarabine
  - Cladribine
  - Pentostatin → *inhibits* the enzyme *adenosine deaminase*
  - It is used to treat *hairy cell leukemia*
- **Pyrimidine:**
  - 5-Fluorouracil [5-FU]
  - Capecitabine

  → **Thymidylate synthase inhibitor**

  - Cytarabine → DNA polymerase inhibitor
  - Gemcitabine → Ribonucleotide reductase inhibitor

  → **Incorporates in DNA**

  - Decitabine
  - Azacitidine or 5-azacytidine
  - Zebularine

  → **Hypomethylating_agent (inhibits DNA methylation)**
- **Raltitrexed – Specific inhibitor of thymidylate synthase**
- **Lometrexol – Inhibits purine synthesis** [inhibits Glycinamide Ribonucleotide Formyltransferase (GARFT)]
- **Pemetrexed –** Used in **pleural mesothelioma** and **non-small cell lung cancer**
- **GnRH agonist:**
  - Leuprore**lin**
  - Gosere**lin**
- **GnRH antagonist:**
  - Ganire**lix**
  - Abare**lix**
- Eagle effect, Eagle phenomenon, or paradoxical zone phenomenon—benzylpenicillin catericide maximum effect at 4 times MIC > then that decreases
- **Braking phenomenon : Diuretics ↓ → ECF ↓ → RBF ↑ → Renin ↓ → Na excretion**

- Chronic administration of loop diuretics results in a diminished natriuretic effect
- Bleomycin—Antibiotic—G_2 specific
- Epipodophyllotoxins:
  - Etoposide
  - Teniposide
- Camptothecin:
  - Topotecan
  - Irinotecan
- Chlorambucil → spares myelocytes—not in AML
- Vincristine → spares Bone Marrow (BM)
- Cisplatin → Maximum nausea and vomiting
  Nephrotoxic, Neurotoxic, Ototoxic.
- Carboplatin → Bone Marrow (BM) toxicity
- Oxaliplatin → Neurotoxicity
- Cyclophosphamide ← Hemorrhagic cystitis
- Ifosfamide ← Syndrome of Inappropriate AntiDiuretic Hormone secretion (SIADH)
- Cladribine → Hairy Cell Leukemia (HCL)
- Langerhans Cell Histiocytosis (LCH)
- Fludarabine → Chronic Lymphocytic Leukemia (CLL)
- Cisplatin + paclitaxel → Cervix Carcinoma
- Alkylating agent → Chronic Leukemia
- Antimetabolites → Acute Leukemia
- Sorafenib → Thyroid Carcinoma
- Sorafenib → HepatoCellular Carcinoma (HCC)
- Sunitinib → Renal Cell Carcinoma (RCC)
- Cisplatin → Larynx, Head and Neck
- Dacarbazine → Melanoma
- Gemcitabine → Pancreatic cancer
- Streptozotocin → Insulinoma
- Interferon (INF)
- Kaposi → liposomal doxorubicin
- Liposomal daunorubicin
- Colorectal cancer → FOLFOX:
  - FOL: Folinic acid (leucovorin)
  - F: Fluorouracil (5-FU)
  - OX: Oxaliplatin (Eloxatin) + Bevacizumab

  (Or)
- FOLFIRI:
  - FOL: Folinic acid (leucovorin)
  - F : Fluorouracil (5-FU)
  - IRI: Irinotecan (Camptosar) + Bevacizumab

- Cyclophosphamide
- Hydroxydaunorubicin [Doxorubicin]
- Oncovin (Vincristine)
- Prednisone or Prednisolone

→ CHOP–R regimen → Non-Hodgkin's Lymphoma (NHL)

- Rituximab
- Adriamycin [Doxorubicin/Hydroxydaunorubicin]
- Bleomycin
- Vinblastine and
- Dacarbazine

→ ABVD regimen ↓ Hodgkin Lymphoma (HL)

- Epirubicin
- Cisplatin
- Fluorouracil (5FU)

→ ECF regimen → advanced Gastric Carcinoma

- Cyclophosphamide
- Methotrexate
- Fluorouracil

→ CMF regimen → Breast Carcinoma

- Cyclophosphamide
- Hydroxydaunorubicin [Doxorubicin]
- Oncovin (Vincristine)
- Prednisone or Prednisolone
- Dactinomycin + Methotrexate → Chorionic Carcinoma

→ CHOP regimen → Gastric Lymphoma (DLBCL)

- Bleomycin
- Etoposide
- Carboplatin

→ BEC regimen → Testicular cancer

- 5-Fluorouracil (5-FU) → Gastrointestinal Tract (GIT) Cancers
- Leiomyosarcoma → Adriamycin (Doxorubicin)
- Mitomycin → Antibiotic with alkylating property
- Bleomycin → Antibiotic but also arrests the cell cycle at the G2 phase
- Estramustine → Alkylating property but also arrests the cell cycle at the M phase
- Bortezomib + lenalidomide + Dexamethasone → Multiple myeloma
- Leflunomide → Disease-Modifying Antirheumatic Drug (DMARD)
- Inhibits the mitochondrial enzyme *dihydroorotate dehydrogenase* used in Polyoma BK Virus Nephropathy
- Levamisole → used in pediculosis and colon cancer
  Effective in steroid—dependent nephrotic syndrome
- Calcineurin inhibitor → downregulates the expression of interleukin 2 (IL-2)
  - Cyclosporine
  - Tacrolimus (also FK-506) → no hirsutism and no gum hypertrophy
- *Glucocorticoids* markedly *decreased IL-1*
- mTOR inhibitor → Sirolimus → ↓ platelet and ↑ lipid
- Everolimus

→ Contraindicated in newborns and G6PD deficiency

- K_1 → phylloquinone, phytomenadione, (from Diet) MC used or phytonadione
- K_2 → menaquinones (from intestinal bacterial flora)

- $K_3 \rightarrow$ menadione (Synthetic)
- INR > 5 – give Vitamin K
- INR > 20 – give FFP
- Unfractioned Heparin – X_a and II_a

→ *(10a and 2a)*

- Low Molecular Weight Heparin (LMWH) – only X_a *(only 10a)*
- Sildenafil: Phosphodiesterase 5, 6 inhibitor (PDE5, 6) s/e includes changes in vision
- β blocker↓: ↑HDL, TGL

VASOMOTOR REVERSAL OF DALE

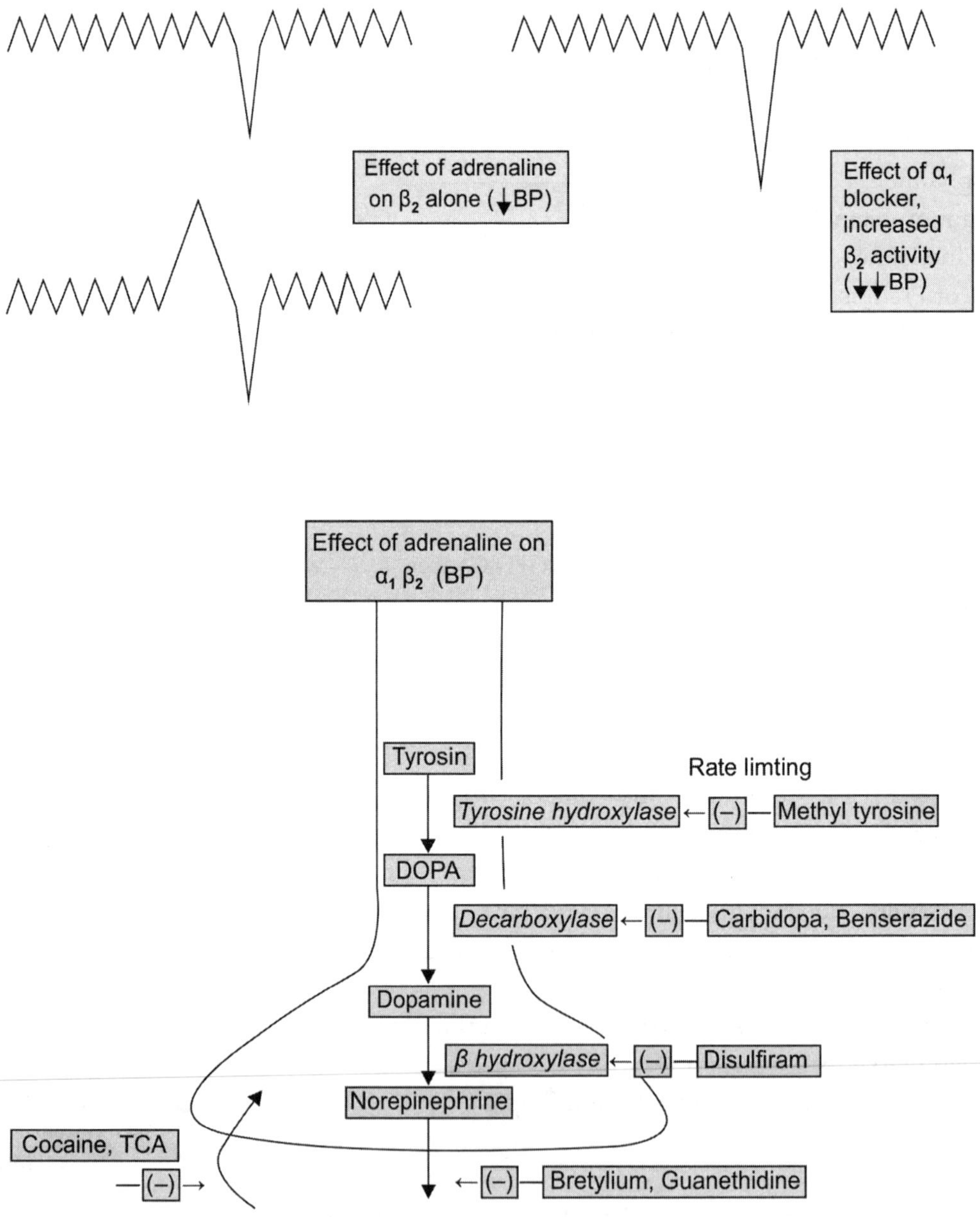

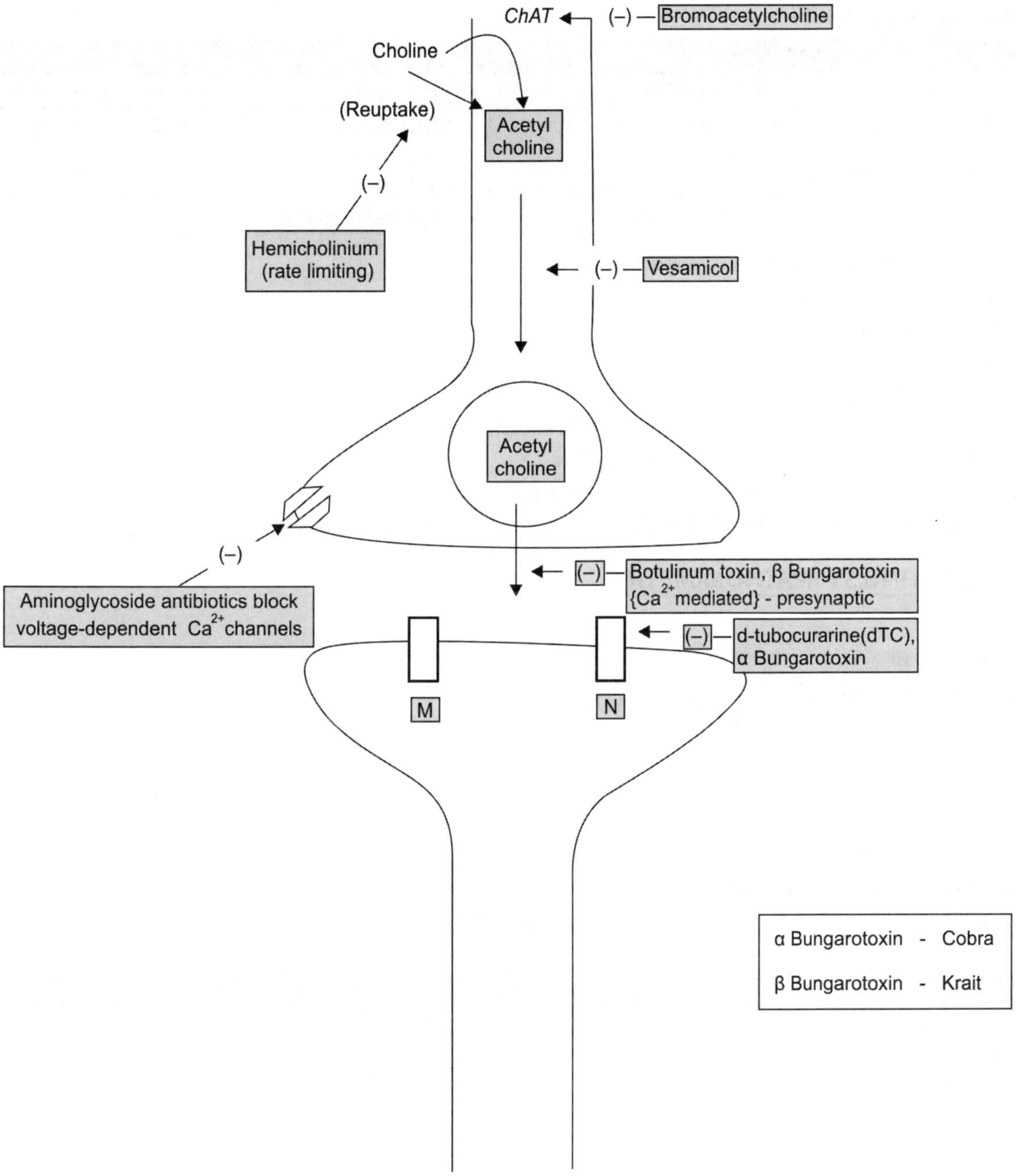

- **ω – Conotoxin (Ziconotide):** Blocks N-type voltage-dependent calcium channels and it is 1000 times that of morphine
- **α – Latrotoxin:** ↑Na^+ Channel, Ach release, paralysis (black widow spider)
- **Thiocyanate:** Inhibitor of Na^+ I^- pump (sodium-iodide symporter)
- **Perchlorate:** ↓Iodide trap
- **Carbachol:** Maximum nicotinic activity
- **Bethanechol:** Minimum nicotinic activity

- **Anticholinesterase inhibitors:**

Group	Properties	Examples	Site
I	• Reversible, Short-Acting	• Edrophonium	• Anionic site
II	• Carbamylating Agents: Intermediate	• Physostigmine • Neostigmine	• Both Anionic and Ester site
III	• Phosphorylating Agents: Long-Duration	• OPC • Organophosphates	• Ester site

- **Oxime** (Obidoxime, Pralidoxime) → **Both sites**
- **Acetylcholine alone**: vasodilator - ↓BP (M_3 endothelium)
- **Acetylcholine** with **Atropine** - ↑BP
- Atropine initially ↓HR – Presynaptic M_2
- **Preganglionic always Acetylcholine**
- **Hyoscine/Scopolamine → Twilight sleep; truth serum**
- **Inocybe/clitocybe** → specific antidote is **atropine**
- **Amanita muscaria** → management: **benzodiazepine**
- **Amanita galerina and amanita phalloides:** Silibinin, penicillin, thioctic acid.

INDIRECTLY ACTING SYMPATHOMIMETICS

- Tyramine
- Methylphenidate
- Pemoline (hepatotoxicity)
- Atomoxetine
- Amphetamine
- Modafinil

(Pemoline, Atomoxetine, Amphetamine, Modafinil → used in ADHD)

- Guanabenz
- Guanoxabenz

(Guanabenz, Guanoxabenz → α_2 agonist)

- **Floppy iris syndrome: Tamsulosin**
- **Pilocarpine, cevimeline: Used in the treatment of dry mouth**

GOUT

Acute Gout	Chronic Gout
• **Only NSAIDs** (except Aspirin as it increases Uric acid) • **Colchicine** • **Steroids**	• Allopurinol • Rasburicase • Febuxostat • Uricosurics

Smoking

- Mecamylamine (nicotinic antagonist)
- Varenicline (nicotinic agonist-partial)
- Buprenorphine
- Amfebutamone
- Clonidine {Cigarette}
- Rimonabant
- Topiramate
- Nortriptyline
- Glucose
- Tryptophan

IMPOTENCE/Erectile dysfunction (ED)

- Sildenafil
- Apomorphine (dopamine receptor agonist)
- Bromomorphine
- Phentolamine
- Ketanserin
- Trazodone
- Alprostadil
- Aviptadil
- Thymoxamine
- Naltrexone
- α_2 adrenergic receptor antagonist: Yohimbine
- Idazoxan

ALCOHOL

- Tretament for dependence
- Naltrexone
- Acamprosate
- Disulfiram
- Benzodiazepine
- Topiramate
- Ondansetron
- Fluoxetine
- **Naltrexone is used in all except for smoking cessation**

HEROIN

- β adrenergic receptor antagonist
- Clonidine
- Methadone: Decrease craving
- Buprenorphine: Decrease craving
- Naltrexone: Decrease relapse (not craving)
- Levomethadyl
- Lofexidine: An α_2A-adrenergic receptor agonist
- **GLP analogue (glucagon-like peptide-1 agonist):**
  - Exenatide
  - Liraglutide
- **Amylin analogue:** Pramlintide
- **DPP: 4 (dipeptidyl peptidase-4) inhibitor:**
  - Sitagliptin
  - Vildagliptin
- Glibenclamide = Glyburide
- **Most potent glucocorticoid:** Betamethasone
- **Maximum glucocorticoid activity:** Dexamethasone
- **Most potent mineralocorticoid:** Fludrocortisone
- **Maximum mineralocorticoid activity:** Aldosterone
- **Least potent glucocorticoid:** Cortisone

- ZERO **mineralocorticoid activity:** Dexamethasone, Betamethasone, Triamcinolone, Methylprednisolone
- ZERO **glucocorticoid activity:** DOCA - deoxycorticosterone acetate
  - **Glucocorticoid with maximum mineralocorticoid activity:** hydrocortisone
- Estrane: 'e +' – androgenic → 19 C
- Gonane: 'e S' – decr. Androgen → 19 C

- Pregnane: 'm, p' – androgenic → 21 C
- Drospirenone has antimineralocorticoid properties
- Tetracycline
- Sparflox (Sparfloxacin): QT interval prolongation
- Mefloquine → Prophylaxis
- Proguanil → Prophylaxis
- Chloroquine → Prophylaxis
- Doxycycline
- Secnidazole: Longest acting
- Satranidazole: No metallic taste

Nitazoxanide

- Giardia
- Cryptosporidium
- Hymenolepis
- Pseudomonas enterocolitica
- Rotavirus

Sleeping sickness

Trypanosoma brucei	Gambiense	Rhodesiense
	• Pentamidine • Eflornithine (abn. CSF)	• Suramin • Melarsoprol

Chagas

- Nifurtimox
- Benznidazole

Balantidium

Tetracycline

- *Leishmaniasis*

• Skin • Sodium stibogluconate
• Visceral • Liposomal amphotericin B • IV antimony • Paromomycin • Sitamaquine • Miltefosine

- **Isospora** → **Cotrimoxazole** (sulfamethoxazole + trimethoprim)
- **Cyclospora** → **Cotrimoxazole** (sulfamethoxazole + trimethoprim)

- **Cryptosporidium** → Nitazoxanide
  Paromomycin
- **Microsporidia** → Fumagillin
  Albendazole
- **Guinea worm** → Metronidazole
- **Liver fluke (fasciola hepatica)** → Triclabendazole
- **Strongyloides: Ivermectin**
- Ciprofloxacin
- Pefloxacin
- Polymyxin
- Colistin
  (Ciprofloxacin, Pefloxacin, Polymyxin, Colistin) → Pseudomonas
- Lumefantrine: Antimalarial drug
- Pyronaridine
- Niclosamide: Taenia solium
- Cefepime: Not against anaerobe

Phenytoin

- Dupuytren's contracture
- Vestibular toxicity
- Vitamin K and D deficiency
- BZD: GABA facilitator
- Barbiturates: GABA mimetic and facilitatory
  Ca^{2+} (absence)
- Valproate
- Ethosuximide
- Lamotrigine (× glutamate release)
- Trimethadione
- Felbamate (NMDA block)
- Tigabine × reuptake (increase GABA)
- GABA transaminase:
  - Valproate
  - Vigabatrin
- Increased release:
  - Gabapentin
  - Pregabalin
- Topiramate
- Felbamate
- SSRI
  (Topiramate, Felbamate, SSRI) → Weight loss
- Valproate →↑ NH_3: Carnitine deficiency
- N-acetylglutamate
- Meperidine: Mydriasis (resemble like atropine)
- (pethidine) Seizures
- GABA agonist—Muscimol
- GABA antagonist—Bicuculline (inhibitor)
- Flurazepam—Long-acting drug
- Flunitrazepam—Date rape drug

Benzodiazepines

- **STOLE** → **S**hort acting: **T**riazolam, **T**emazepam, **O**xazepam, **L**orazepam and **E**stazolam (used in insomnia)
- **CADOL** → **C**hlordiazepoxide, **A**lprazolam, **D**iazepam, **O**xazepam and **L**orazepam (as antianxiety)
- **Ramelteon** →↑ prolactin and ↓TSH
- **Akinesia:** Rx — **Apomorphin** (D_4 agonist) (off period)
- **Restless leg syndrome: Ropinirole**
- **Levodopa: D_2**
- Postural hypotension (D_1)
- Hypertension (α_1)
- Nausea, Vomiting — (Rx – Domperidone)
- Mydriasis (α_1)—Contraindicated in Acute Congestive Glaucoma (ACG)
- Psychosis — (Rx – quetiapine, clozapine)
- **Antipsychotics: ↓D_1**
- Sedation
- Antiemetic (anticholinergics)
- Weight gain
- Postural hypotension (α block)
- D_2 block—extrapyramidal symptoms, seizure (atypical)
- ↑Prolactin
- Acetyl L Carnitine →
  - Ach analogue
  - Antioxidant

Alzheimer disease

- **Huntington's**
- **Rx: D_2 block:**
  - Chlorpromazine
  - Haloperidol
- Olanzapine
- **Dopamine depletion:** Tetrabenazine
- Reserpine

ERGOT	NON-ERGOT
• Bromocriptine • Pergolide	• Ropinirole • Ramipexole • Rotigotine • Sumanirole

- **Topiramate—Weight loss**

Na Channel block

- Phenytoin
- Carbamazepine
- Valproate
- Topiramate
- Lamotrigine
- Lacosamide (CRMP-2 block: {collapsin-response mediator protein-2} → Partial seizure)
- Zonisamide

- **Lacosamide → In Partial seizure by CRMP-2block: {collapsin-response mediator protein-2}**
  - Felbamate → Inhibitor of NMDA
  - Topiramate → Inhibition of GluR5 ***kainate*** receptors

  (Felbamate, Topiramate) → Weight loss

  Weight loss could represent a key mechanism

Lenox gastaut: Lamotrigene, rufinamide
WEST syndrome: ACTH
Infantile spasm: Vigabatrin > ACTH > ganaxolone Vigabatrin ↓ (with Tuberous Sclerosis); ACTH → (WEST syndrome)
Absence seizures: • < 3 years: Ethosuximide • > 3 years: Valproate
Rolandic epilepsy: Carbamazepine (CBZ)
Catamanial epilepsy: Ganaxolone ↓ (Infantile spasm)
Gilles de Tourette: Haloperidol, Guanfacine, Pimozide
Janz syndrome: Juvenile myoclonic epilepsy (JME) - valproate

Could represent a key mechanism

- **Thioridazine**
- ↓extrapyramidal symptoms (EPS↓) (antipsychotics)
- ↑anticholinergic (but no antiemesis)
- ↑α - block
- **Olanzapine:** Weight gain
- **Clozapine:** Block $5HT_{2A}$, D_2, D_4
- **(antisuicide)** agranulocytosis
- Seizure
- Paradoxical sialorrhea
- **Aripiprazole:** Partial agonist $5HT_{1A}$ and D_2 antagonist $5HT_{2A}$

Lithium:

Lithium↑	Lithium↓
	NSAID
carbonic anhydrase inhibitors (CAI)	Tetracycline
xanthine	thiazides

- **Sydenham: Carbamazepine (cbz), Valproate, Haloperidol**

  (Carbamazepine, Valproate) → **(Severe)**
- μ_1 **– Supraspinal: Analgesia, euphoric, depression.**
- μ_2 **– spinal: Analgesia, Respiratory depression, constipation**
- **Pethidine**
  - → ↑Seizure ----- Norpethidine
  - → ↓**Seizure** ----- **Anesthetic** (by α_2 reuptake)
- **Tizanidine:** α_2 agonist – muscle relaxant
- Sulfenatyl: Most potent – truncal rigidity.

  The cause is unknown, but restless leg syndrome is especially common among pregnant women and also among uremic or diabetic patients with neuropathy.

Teratogenicity

ACE inhibitor: Renal damage
Carbamazepine: Neural tube defects
Ethanol: Fetal alcohol syndrome
Iodide: Goitre
Isotretinoin: CNS, Face and Ear malformation
Lithium: Ebsein's anomaly
Misoprostol: Mobius syndrome
Penicillamine: Cutis laxa
Phenytoin: Fetal hydantoin syndrome
Streptomycin: 8th nerve damage
Terracycline: Discoloration of teeth
Thalidomide: Phocomelia
Valproic acid: Chondrodysplasia (Contradi syndrome)

CHAPTER 9

Forensic Medicine

LAWS AND SECTIONS

IPC	Content
324 326 IPC	Dangerous weapon
319	Hurt
320	Grievous hurt
325	Punishment of grievous hurt
51	Oath
82	Child < 7 yrs not punishable
83	Child >7 yrs maybe punishable
84	McNaughton's rule
85	Involuntary intoxication
86	Voluntary intoxication
87–90	Consent
88-93	Legal protection of doctors
191	Perjury
193	Punishment of perjury
299	Culpable homicide
300	Murder
302	Punishment of murder
304	Punishment of culpable homicide
304A	Criminal negligence
304B	Dowry death
306	Abetment of suicide
307	Attempt murder
308	Attempt culpable homicide
309	Attempt suicide for 1 yr
312–316	Injury to unborn/born child
318	Concealment of birth
330	Torture
351	Assault
354	Outrage of modesty—force

Contd…

Contd…

IPC	Content
509	Outrage of modesty word/gesture
359–369	Kidnapping
375, 376	Rape
377	Unnatural sex
497	Adultery
498	Detaining married women
498A	Husband/relative subjecting torture
503	Criminal intimidation
510	Misconduct by drunken in public
511	Attempt to commit offence

CrPC	Content
39	Citizen bound to inform
53	Examination without consent
54	Accused voluntary examination
160	Summon by police
174	Police inquest
162	Statement received by police
176	Magistrate inquest
161	Examination by police
61–69	Summon

Year	Act
1912	Indian Lunacy Act
1987	Mental Health Act
1956	Indian Medical Council Act
1986	COPRA/Juvenile Justice Act
1994	Organ Transplantation Act, Prenatal sex determination
1940	Drugs and Cosmetics Act
1971	MTP Act
1985	Narcotic Drugs and Psychotropic Substances Act
1998	Biomedical waste management

Age (in years)	Importance
5	The Railways Act
< 7	Not responsible for criminal activity
< 10	Kidnapping
> 12	Consent
14	Factories Act
< 15	Rape even wife

Contd…

Contd...

Age (in years)	Importance
< 16	Rape of women
18	Marriage age for women, consent for act likely to harm
21	Marriage age for men, major
25	MP/MLA
35	President

Contusion

Blue	Deoxy hb	Day 1
Brown	Hemosiderin	Day 3
Green	Hematoin	Day 6
Yellow	Bilirubin	> 1 week
Normal	> 2 weeks	

Blood Analysis

Chemical

- Benzidine test
- Phenolphthalein test (Kastle-Mayer test)
- Leucomalachite green test
- Orthotolidine test
- Guaiacum test.

Microscopic Test

- Teichmann—Hemin crystals
- Takayama—Hemochromatin
- Spectroscopic test—more reliable
- Acid elution inhibition test
- Precipitin test—animal/human blood.

SEMEN

Florence test	Choline	No false negative but false positive
Barberio test	Spermine	Negative in azoospermia
Creatinine phosphokinase	> 400 μ/mL	Diagnostic
Acid phosphatase	Confirm with tartaric acid	

Heavy Metals

- Harrison and Gilroy test
- Neutron activation analysis
- Atomic absorption spectroscopy
- Flameless atomic absorption spectroscopy
- Paraffin/dermal nitrate test = gunpowder.

Rules and Principles

Locard's exchange principle	Transfer of material between two when they come in contact
Puppe's rule	One fracture line prevents other fracture
Quetelet's rule	Biological variation

Gustafson Formula—SCRAPT

- Secondary dentition
- Cementum
- Root eruption
- Attrium
- Periodontal
- Transparency of root*

Gettler test: Chloride containing heart in drowning

Karl Pearson's formula: Stature

Bertillium system: Anthropometry

McNaughton's rule/Durham's/Curren's rule: Criminal responsibility of insane

Casper dictum: Time since death

- Air:Water:Earth—1:2:8 (decomposition)

Nystens rule: Rigor mortis not starts in all muscles simultaneously.

Infanticide

- Raygets hydrostatic test
- Forders static test—wt of lung double after respiration
- Ploquert test
- Breslows second life test—stomach with gases
- Wredin test—middle ear changes after birth.

Alcohol

- Alcohol dehydrogenase
- Breath analyzer
- Cavett test
- Gas chromatography
- Kozelka test.

Racial Indices

- Cephalic index
- Brachial index
- Crural index
- Radio/tibio
- Humero/femoral index
- Nasal index.

Cephalic index = max width of skull/max length of skull × 100

Indices for Sex

- Ischiopubic index
- Corporobasal index
- Sacral index
- Sternal index
- Sciatic notch
- Medullary index.

Racial Featues of Skull

Aryans and Negroes	70–74.9	Dolicocephaly
Europeans and Chinese	75–79.9	Mesaticephaly
Mongoleans	80–84.9	Brachycephaly

Fingerprint Patterns: Most Common

Loop > whorls > arch > composite

Temporary teeth (20)	Month
Lower central incisor	6
Upper central incisor	7
Upper lateral incisor	8
Lower lateral incisor	9
First molar	1 year
Canine	1-and-a-half years
Second molar	2 years

Permanent teeth (32)	Age of eruption
First molar	6
Central incisor	7
Lateral incisor	8
First premolar	9
Second premolar	10
Canine	11
Second molar	12—14
Third molar	17–25

Terms with Meanings

Lynching	Public hanging
Mugging (choke holding)	Strangulation against forearm
Garroting	Ligature over neck tightened quickly
Bansdola	Neck compressed between two sticks
Burking	Smothering+traumatic asphyxia
Choking	Occlusion of internal air passage
Smothering	Occlusion of external air passage

Contd...

Contd...

Gagging	Filling cloth in mouth
Trottling	Manual strangulation
Falanga	Beating on sole
El Telefono	Beating of both ears
El Quirofano	Beating on abdomen
Cattle prod	Electric shock
Placana	Electric wire in vagina, anus, nipple, testes
Black salve	Heat material in anus
Dry submarine	Tying plastic bag over face
Wet submarine	Forced immersion in water
Labandera	Suspension by wrist
Mercelago	Suspension by ankle
El Planton	Prolonged standing
El Cabellete	Forced straddling of a bar
Parrot perch	Like parrot hang
Chepuwa	Tight clamping both thighs with bamboo

PERVETED SEX

Sadism	Infliction of pain on partner
Masochism	Infliction of pain on self
Sadism + masochis	Bondage
Necrophilia (297 IPC)	Intercourse with dead/dying victim
Fetichism	Gratification by contact with fetish objects
Transvestism/Eonism	Wearing clothes of opp sex
Uranism	Gratification by fingering, fellatio, cunnilingus
Sin of Gomorrah	Fellatio/cunnlingus
Voyeurism/peeping toms/scotophilic	Watching sexual act
Troluism	Perveted husband watching wife with others
Frotteurism	Rubbing genitalia against others
Urolangia/Coprophilia	Sight/odor of feces/urine
Lesbianism/tribadism	Female homosexuality
Sodomy/buggery/Greek love	Anal sex
Bestiality	With animal
Incest	With close relatives

Mummification

- Increased temperature
- Decreased moisture
- Air circulation
- Arsenic/antimony.

Saponification

- Warm temperature
- Humid
- Decreased air
- Cl perfringens
- Unsaturated fatty acid to saturated fatty acid.

Lividity

CO	Cherry red
Cyanide	Pink/red
H_2S	Greenish blue
Phosphorus	Dark brown
Nitrate	Reddish brown/blue
Chlorate	Chocolate brown
Opium	Black

No Activated Charcoal—CHACH

- Cyanide
- Heavy metal
- Alcohol
- Corrosive poison
- Hydrocarbon.

No Hemodialysis

- $CuSO_4$
- BZD
- OPC
- Kerosene
- Digoxin.

Urine

- Carbolic acid—greenish brown
- HNO_3—brown
- Barbiturate—liquid gold
- Amphetamine—liquid gold.

Odor

Zinc phosphide	Fruity odor
H_2S	Rotten egg
Aluminum	Garlic
Arsenic phophide	Garlic
Cyanide	Bitter almond
Kerosene	OPC
Cannabis	Burnt rope

Delayed Putrefaction

- Arsenic
- Zinc chloride
- Carbolic acid.

Poison Trivia

Cholera DDx	Arsenic
GBS	Thallium
Plant viper	Abrus
Plant penicillin	Endrin

Toxicity

- AS_2O_3—Most toxic
- $HgCl_2$—Most toxic
- PbS—Least toxic
- Pb_2O_4—Vermillon.

PCT

- Cadmium
- CCl_4
- Mercury
- Phenol
- Lysol.

Miosis

- Carbolic acid
- CCl_4
- Morphine
- OPC
- Barbiturate.

Carbamates

- Stigmine
- Phonium
- Propoxur
- Carbaryl
- Demacarium
- Donepezil
- Revastigmine.

Embalming

- Phenol
- Methanol
- Formalin
- Mercuric chloride

- Sodium lauryl sulfate
- Eucalyptus oil.

HEROIN NAMES

Brown sugar	Monoacetyl morphine
Heroin	Diacetyl morphine
Speed ball	Cocaine+heroin

Carbon Monoxide

20%	Headache
30 to 40%	Cherry red
50%	Drunkenness
70%	Fatal

Preservation

Carbolic acid	NaCl
All other acid	Rectified spirit
Uric acid	Alcohol
Alcohol	Sodium fluoride, potassium oxalate
Sodium fluoride	Sodium nitrate, potassium oxalate
Oxalic acid	Sodium citrate
Ethylene glycol	Sodium citrate

Bullets

Bullet	Function
Tandem bullet	Piggy back
Dum bum	Expand
Yawning	Irregular
Incendinary	Ignite
Frangible	Color, trailing
Tracer	Ba_2O_2, Mg, Strontium
Tumbling	Rotation
Baton	Rubber
Souvenir	Left in body

Hanging

2 kg	Vein
3 kg	Artery
15 kg	Trachea
20 to 30 kg	Vertebral

PCS—Blackpowder

- Potassium nitrate
- Charcoal
- Sulfur
- Nitrocellulose
- Nitroglycerine
- Nitroguanidine.

Tatooing: Gunpowder

Blackening: Smoke

Burning: Fire

Superfetation: Diff cycle, diff coitus

Superfecundation: Same cycle, diff coitus

Lividity: Appears for half-an-hr, fixed in 6 hrs, merges with putrefaction

Marbling: 36 to 48 hrs

Putrefaction: 12 to 24 hrs—RIF, undersurface of liver

Rigidity: Starts in 1 to 2 hrs, in winter in 1 to 2 days.

Putrefaction: Starts first in larynx/trachea, and last in bone.

Lamps (UV and IR)

Old tattoos	IR photography
Faded tattoos	UV lamp
Dried semen	UV lamp

Postmortem Caloricity

- Sunstroke
- Pontine hemorrhage
- Tetanus
- Strychnine
- Severe acute bacterial viral infection.

Height

- Humerus × 5
- Femur × 4
- Spine × 3.

CHAPTER 10

Social and Preventive Medicine

DEMOGRAPHIC CYCLE

Stage	Name	Birth	Death
1	High stationary	Increasing	Increasing
2	Early expanding	Stable	Decreasing
3	Late expanding	Decreasing	More decreasing
4	Low stationary	Decreasing	Decreasing
5	Declining	B < D	

Person	Significance
John Snow	Father of public health
Lord Dawson	Concept of health centre
Todd Commission	Community med dep in England
Jules Guerin	Coined social medicine
Neuman and Virchow	Social medicine
John Snow	Father of epidemiology, cholera study in London
James Lind	Scurvy
McMahon Pugh	Web of causation
Reed	Yellow fever
Goldberger	Pellagra
John M Last	Defined epidemiology
Hippocrates	Father of medicine, oath, first true epidemiologist
Sydenham	First distinguished epidemiologist
Samuel Hahnemann	Homeopathy
Pettenkofer	Multifactorial causation
Morgagni	Pathologic anatomy
Germany	Sickness inclusion
Russia	Socialized medicine

Disease

Control	Ceases to be a public health problem
Elimination	Large geographical area
Eradication	All or none, whole world

7 April 1948: World Health Day.

India: July 1

Tropical Diseases

- Malaria
- Filaria
- Leishmaniasis
- Schistosoma
- Trypanosomes
- Leprosy.

Kuppuswamy Index

- Education
- Occupation
- Income.

Holingshead Index (USA)

- Education
- Occupation
- Residential address.

Night blindness	> 1 %
Bitot spots	> 0.5%
Corneal xerosis	> 0.01%
Corneal ulcer	> 0.05%

Anemia: WHO

6 mths–6 yrs	11 gm/dL
6 yrs–14 yrs	12 gm/dL
Adult male	13 gm/dL
Adult female	12 gm/dL

Nutrition Formulae

Protein Efficiency Ratio: Weight increase in gram/gram of protein consumed

NPU: Retained nitrogen/nitrogen in food

Biological value: Retained nitrogen/absorbed nitrogen.

STEPS: Risk factor surveillance of chronic non communicable diseases

IDEAS: Measure quantity of disability in mental disorder

- Self-care
- Interpersonal activities
- Communication and understanding
- Work.

ICIDH: International Classification of Impairment, Disability and Handicap

ICF: International Classification of Functional disability, health.

Killer Bacteriae

- Cholera
- Typhoid
- Plague
- Pertussis.

POLIO

- Most common paralytic polio
- Good antigen
- Vaccine-induced polio.

DEMOGRAPHIC TRIVIA

Measles elimination	< 1/million
Leprosy	< 1 in one lakh
Vaccine-induced encephalitis (DPT)	1 in 40000
Vaccine-induced polio	1 in 2.5 million
Same fingerprint	1 in 64 million

Mental Retardation

IQ	MR
50–79	Mild
35–49	Moderate
20–34	Severe
< 20	Profound

Vaccines Contraindicated in Pregnancy

- BCG
- MMR
- Varicella
- Yellow fever
- JE
- IPV.

Killer Viruses

- Rabies
- Hepatitis B
- Influenza B
- JE
- KFD.

SCALES

Visual analogue scale	Pain
Likert scale	Response to equation strongly negative to strongly positive
Guttman scale	Increasing strong expression

COMMITTEES

Committee	Recommendations
Bhore	3 months SPM posting, PHC, social physician
Mudaliar	Strengthening PHC
Chadha	Multipurpose worker
Mukherjee	Family planning asst
Jungalwalla	Private practice
Kartar Singh	Committee on multipurpose worker, subcentre, health supervisor
Shrivastav	Medical education, paraprofessional workers (teacher, postmaster), referral service
Rural Health Scheme	Medical College, PHC

NGOs

Name	Disease
Hind Kushtt Nivaran Sangh	Leprosy
Bharat Sevak Samaj	Sanitation
Central Social Welfare Board	Women and children
Kasturba Memorial Fund	Women
Rockfeller Foundation	Hookworm, Borehole, virology institute of public health
FORD Foundation	RCA—Reasearch cum action, rural health and family welfare

Screening time: First possible point to final critical diagnosis

Lead time: First possible point to usual time of diagnosis (**advantage gained by screening**)

API > 5: Mass treatment

API < 2: No presumptive treatment, focal spraying

API > 2: Susceptibility test

Eligible couple: 15 to 45 years.

Some Important Numbers

20 spots/sq inch = tourniquet test

150/sq ft = mosquito net

1 in 3500 = doctor

1 in 5000 = nurse

Extra calories

Pregnancy = 300 kcals

Lactation < 6 mths = 550 kcals

> 6 mths = 400 kcals

Vitamin A

1 IU = 0.3 micrograms
6 microgram beta carotene = 1 microgram retinol equivalent

CEREALS

Rice	High lysine
Wheat	Low lysine and threonine
Jawar and Bajra	Low lysine and threonine
Maize	High leucine, low lysine tryptophan
Pulses	Low cysteine, and low methionine

Water-related Vector

1. Yellow fever
2. Onchocerca
3. Gambisian sleeping sickness
4. Pollutants.

Propagative: Plague in rat flea

Cyclopropagative: Malaria in mosquito

Cyclodevelopmental: Filaria/guinea worm

Hyperendemic: High incidence/prevalence and all ages affected

Holoendemic: Children affected at high rates, adults show less.

Bioterrorism

Category A only

- Anthrax
- Plague
- Botulinium
- Tularemia
- Small pox
- Viral hemorrhagic fever.

Definitions

Incubation period: Invasion of agent to appearance of first sign/symptom

Latent period: Disease initiation to disease detection

Serial interval: Time taken from primary case to secondary case

Generation time: Receipt of infection by host to period of maximal infectivity

Secondary attack rate: No. of individuals susceptible to disease who develop it after exposure excluding primary case within the first incubation period

Quarantine: Limitation of freedom of a person suspected to be infected, not longer than incubation period.

Isolation: Separation for period of communicability

Measles	3 days
Chicken pox, herpes zoster, diphtheria, influenza	6 days
Hepatitis A, TB (with treatment)	3 weeks
Mumps	Swelling subsides
Pertussis	5 days after erythromycin
Shigella, salmonella	3 consecutive negative stool culture
Plague	48 hrs
Meningococcus	1 day after treatment

Personality	Contribution
Von Pirquet	Tuberculin test
Louis Pasteur	Germ theory Sterilization Coined term vaccine Anthrax, rabies vaccine
Robert koch	TB, Cholera, staining technique
Ogston	Staphylococcus
Loeffler	Diphtheria
Nicolaier	Tetanus
Fraenkel	Pneumococcus
Hoffmann	Syphilis
Bleferink	Coined virus
Luska	Electron microscope
Ehlrich	Acid-fast stain

OILS

PUFA	Safflower oil
MUFA	Groundnut oil
Saturated fatty acid	Coconut oil
Linoleic acid	Safflower oil
Linolenic acid	Soyabean oil
Archidonic acid	Meat, egg, milk
Eicosapentanoic acid	Fish oil

Midarm Circumference

> 13.5 = Normal
12.5–13.5 = Mild to moderate malnutrition
< 12.5 = Severe malnutrition

Disease	Crop	Toxin
Lathyrism	Kesari dal	BOAA
Endemic ascites	Crotalaria (jhunjunia)	Pyrrollizidine
Epidemic dropsy	Argemon Mexicana	Sanguinarine

Gomez's Classification

110–90%	Normal
75–89%	1st degree
60–74%	2nd degree
< 60%	3rd degree

Food Poisoning

1–6 hrs	Staph aureus—milk, salad
6–24 hrs	Cl perfringens—meat, reheated
12–24 hrs	Salmonella—milk, poultry
12–36 hrs	Botulinism—canned food
12–24 hrs	B.cereus—raw dried processed food

Pneumonia

RR

> 60/min— < 2 months

> 50/min— 2–12 months

> 40/min— > 12 months

Severe Pneumonia

- Chest indrawing
- Nasal flaring
- Grunting
- Cyanosis.

Very Severe Pneumonia

- Convulsions
- Coma
- Inability to take food.

Notifiable Diseases

WHO: Louse borne typhus, relapsing fever, polio, malaria, influenza

International health registry: Cholera, plague, yellow fever

FORMULAE

Sullivan index: Life expectancy—(time bed ridden/inabled)
HALE includes time spent in poor health

DALY: No. of years lost due to poor health or death

TDI = (NOAEL or LOAEL)/UF

PQLI includes: IMR, Literacy, life expectancy

HDI includes: Life expectancy at birth, knowledge, Real GDP/capita (PPP)

Where:

NOAEL = No-observed-adverse-effect-level

LOAEL = Lowest-observed-adverse-effect-level

UF = Uncertainty factor

TDI = Tolerable daily intake

GV = TDI × Body wt × P (fraction of tissue Doppler imaging)/C (water consumption)

GV is guideline value

Fecal streptococci in water—recent contamination

Clostridium in water—remote contamination

WASTE MANAGEMENT

1	Human anatomical waste
2	Animal waste
3	Micro and biotech waste
4	Sharps
5	Medicine and cytotoxics
6	Solid waste (blood-stained)
7	Solid waste
8	Liquid waste
9	Incineration ash
10	Chemicals

1, 2, 3, 6 – YELLOW

3, 6, 7 – RED

4, 7 – BLUE

5, 9, 10 – BLACK

Case control	Cohort
Few subjects	Large subjects
Rare disease	Rare exposure
Quick and easy	Long
Different causes	Different diseases
Matching	Comparison
RR/odd's ratio	RR/Attributable risk
No difference between association and cause	Evaluation of therapy

Relative risk = Incidence in exposed/incidence in non exposed × 100

Attributable risk = Incidence in exposed – incidence in non exposed/incidence in exposed × 100

Randomized controlled trial	Nonrandomized controlled trial
Blinding	Uncontrolled
Pilot study	Natural experiment
Bias/attrition	Before and after comparison

Judging Causality

- Temporal association
- Strength of association
- Specificity of association
- Consistency of association
- Biological plausibility
- Coherence of association.

National Health Policy, 2002

- Polio and yaws eradicated
- Leprosy eliminated
- Integrated system of surveillance (above till 2005)
- Zero level HIV/AIDS—2007
- Eliminate filarial—2015, All others by 2010.

CHAPTER 11 Biostatistics

Measurements are made of different types of variables.

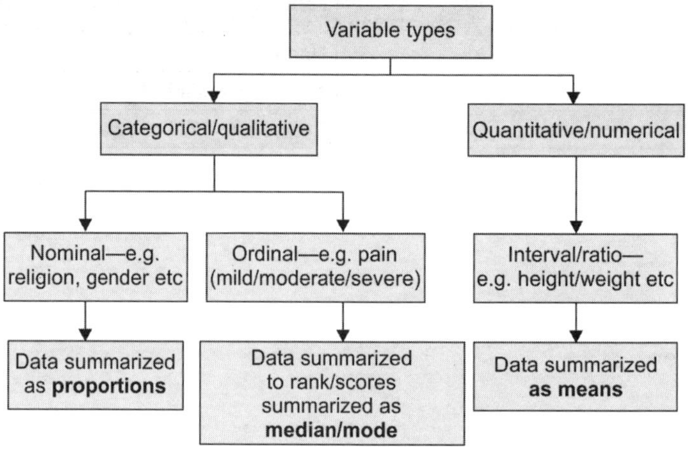

TYPES OF DISTRIBUTIONS

- Normal (Gaussian)

Data symmetrically distributed on both sides of mean
Forms a bell shaped curve in frequency distribution plot

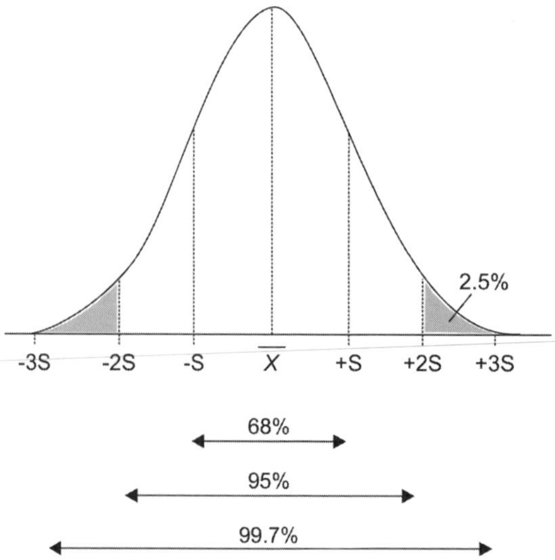

Fig. 11.1: Normal curve

- Non-normal

Data skewed

Bimodal, Poisson

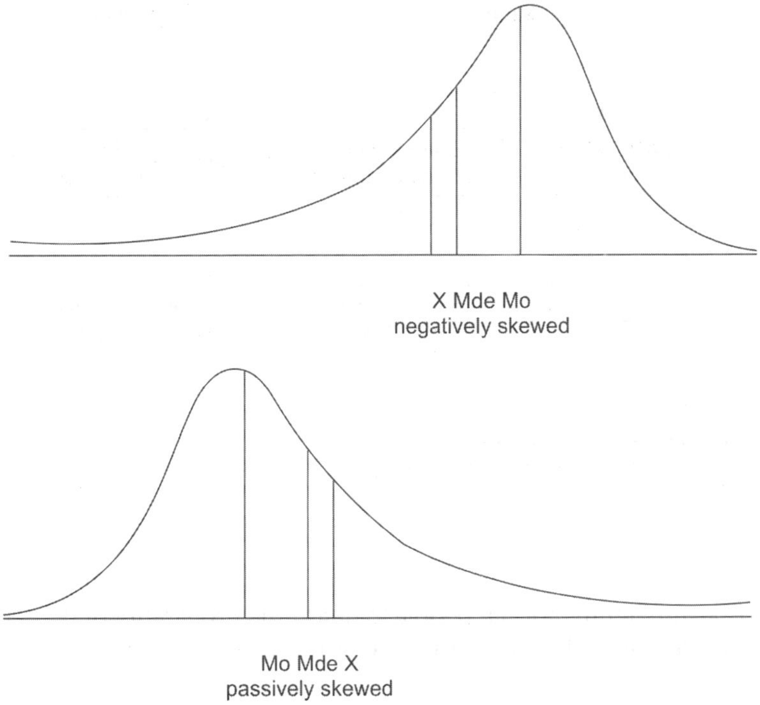

Fig. 11.2: Skewed deviations

Table 11.1: How to choose a statistical test?

		CI				C2	C3
		Comparison				Association of two variables	Regression analysis of two variables
		of 2 data sets		of >2 data sets			
		Paired	Unpaired	Paired	Unpaired		
		C1a	C1b	C1c	C1d		
R1	Normally distributed continuous data (summarized as means)	Paired t test	Unpaired t test	Repeated measures ANOVA	One-way ANOVA	Pearson correlation	Linear regression
R2	Scores, ranks and non-normally distributed continuous data (summarized as medians)	Wilcoxon signed rank test	Wilcoxon rank sum test (Mann-Whitney test)	Friedman test	Kruskal-Wallis test	Spearman's rank correlation	Nonparametric regression
R3	Dichotomous data (summarized as proportions)	McNemar's test	Fisher's test or Chi square test	Cochrane Q	Chi square test	Contingency coefficients	Logistic regression

From 'A Practical Approach to PG Dissertation'

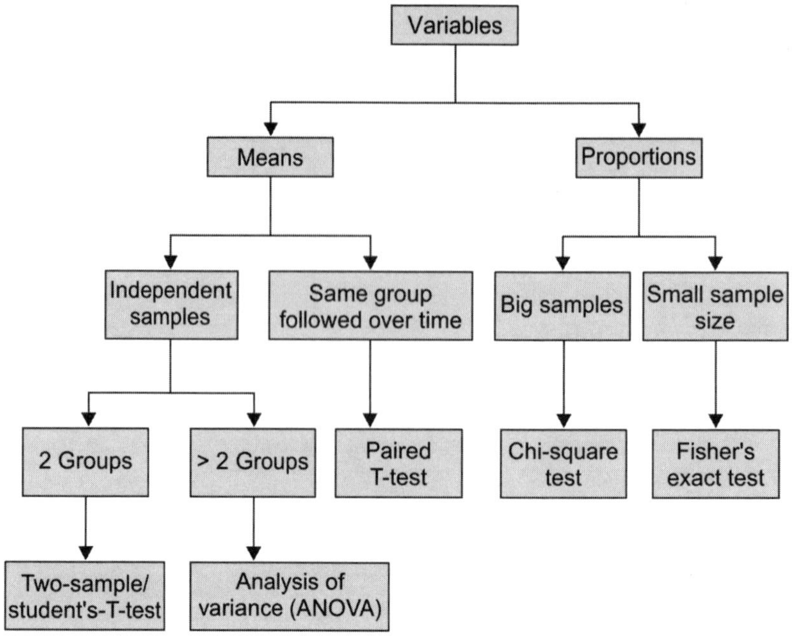

SCREENING TEST

The Screening test is done on apparently normal people to detect the probability of them having the specific health problem. There are 'disease criteria' and 'test criteria' necessary to be satisfied for us to do a particular screening test for a particular disease.

The screening test is not confirmatory and hence:

- A positive test does not mean that the person has the disease definitely
- A negative test does not mean that the person is definitely free of the disease
- So to assess how good a screening test is (Validity), its results have to be compared to a confirmatory/diagnostic test. The following table shows the different possibilities.

	Diagnostic test positive [Diseased]	Diagnostic test negative [Not diseased]
Screening test positive	True positive (a)	False positive (b)
Screening test negative	False negative (c)	True negative (d)

Sensitivity

It is the probability that an individual with the disease will test positive.

The number of patients showing a positive test who really have the disease (TP) divided by all patients who have the disease (TP+FN). A test with high sensitivity will not miss many patients who have the disease (i.e. few false FN).

Specificity

Thus specificity is the probability that an individual without the disease will test negative.

The number of patients showing a negative test and do not have the disease (TN) divided by the number of patients who do not have the disease. A test with high specificity will infrequently identify patients as having a disease when they do not (i.e. few FP sensitivity and specificity are inherent to the test not affected by the prevalence. Likelihood ratios are also independent of prevalence.

Sensitivity and specificity are interdependent. F or a given test, an increase in sensitivity is accompanied by a decrease in specificity and vice versa.

Positive Predictive Value

The likelihood that a patient with a positive test has the disease or the probability that a positive test correctly identifies an individual who actually has the disease.

Negative Predictive Value

NPV represents the likelihood that a patient who has a negative test is free of the disease. It is the probability that a negative test correctly identifies an individual who does not have the disease.

To Summarize

Term	Meaning	Calculation
True positive (TP)	# Patients with the disease who have a positive test result	-
True negative (TN)	# Patients without the disease who have a negative test result	-
False positive (FP)	# Patients without the disease who have a positive test result	-
False negative (FN)	# Patients with the disease who have a negative test result	-
Sensitivity = True positive rate (TPR)	The probability that a patient with the disease will have a positive test result	TP / (TP + FN)
1 - Sensitivity = False-negative rate (FNR)	The probability that a patient with the disease will have a negative test result	FN / (TP + FN)
Specificity = True negative rate (TNR)	The probability that a patient without the disease will have a negative test result	TN / (TN + FP)
1 - Specificity = False-positive rate (FPR)	The probability that a patient without the disease will have a positive test result	FP / (TN + FP)
Positive predictive value	The probability that a patient with a positive test result will have the disease	TP / (TP + FP)
Negative predictive value	The probability that a patient with a negative test result will not have the disease.	TN / (TN + FN)
Accuracy	The probability that the results of a test will accurately predict presence or absence of disease	(TP + TN) / (TP + TN + FP + FN)

It is of importance to note that sensitivity and specificity are inversely proportional to each other. If sensitivity of a test increases specificity reduces and vice versa.

Serial testing – Application of two or more screening tests one after the other. ↑Specificity - ↑PPV*

Parallel testing – Application of two or more screening tests at the same time. ↑ Sensitivity - ↑NPV*

*Predictive values depend on disease prevalence and as such a generalization is difficult to make.

Bias

Selection bias:

- Berksonian bias – using hospital records to estimate population prevalence
- Non responders bias.

Hawthorne effect: Measurement bias - subject behavior altered because they know that they are being studied.

Pgymalion effect: Experimenter expectancy is communicated to the subjects.

Recall bias: Subjects could not remember events accurately.

Ascertainment bias: Misclassification of outcome.

Verification bias: Can be corrected by gold standard test in random samples.

Confounding bias: Problem in selection of risk factors. Confounder is the one related to both disease and exposure. On stratification confounder will have decreased risk.

Lead Time Bias

When treatment is no longer effective after early screening the survival of patient apparently increase without change in overall mortality and natural course of the disease.

Length Time Bias

Early screening test to uncover slowly progressing disease as against rapidly progressing one. Screening test preferentially detects less severe disease and apparently increases the survival time.

Late look bias is a kind of length time bias in which only less severe disease are studied as aggressive forms are missed as the disease kills the patients early.

Reliability

Ability of a test measure the same parameter consistently.

Types

- Inter rater – across observers
- Split half – within the test
- Test and retest – across situations.

Accuracy

- Ability of measuring what is intended.
- *Reliability = Repeatability = Precision = Consistency*
- *Accuracy = Validity.*

Null Hypothesis

The opposite of what actually you intend to show. It says that the results are occurring by chance. Our aim is to defend the null hypothesis .

P-Value

The probability of a result which occurring by the chance. If it p value is ≤ 0.05% it is said to be statistically significant. P value ≤ 0.05% then null hypothesis is rejected.

- It tells only the statistical significance but not the actual clinical significance
- It cannot predict the degree of benefit for a given patient
- Will not tell whether the study is correct or true, but will tell the result has not occurred merely by chance
- P-value of anything below 0.05 is the same. P-value of 0.0004 is not superior to p-value of 0.04.

Confidence Interval

Tells how far the estimates or results from the sample population will lie when extrapolated to the whole population. It is used to generalize the results from the sample studied. Usually the confidence interval is kept as 95%.

If the confidence interval for odds ratio and relative risk contains '1.0' then it is not significant. It should lie in either positive side or negative side.

Type I error: (α-error)

The probability of rejecting null hypothesis when null hypothesis is really true. Alpha error is given by p-value. 5% accepted.

Type II error: (β-error)

The probability of not rejecting null hypothesis when it is actually false. 20% accepted.

	Null Hypothesis True	Null Hypothesis False
Reject	α – error, Type I error	
Fail to reject		β – error, Type II error

Percentile

The percentage of population below a specific value.

Intention to Treat Analysis

Treat as randomized. Avoid cross over and will not be affected by dropouts.

Nominal Variable

- Categorical variable
- Normal distribution
- Poisson distribution
- Known probability of occurring an event occurring or not.

Measures of Central Tendency

- Mean – average of all observations
- Median – observation that divides the data into two halves exactly when arranged in order of smallest to largest.
- Mode – most frequent event.

Measures of Dispersion

- Range
- Standard error of mean
- Standard deviation.

Kaplan-Meier Analysis

Kaplan-Meier analysis measures the ratio of surviving patients divided by the total number of patients at risk

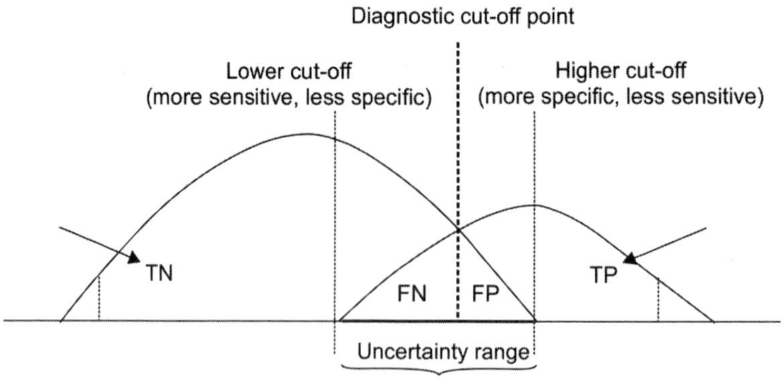

For example, if the cut-off is moved to the right, then the false positives will decrease; hence the positive predictive value increases.

CHAPTER 12

ENT

COCHLEA CROSS-SECTION

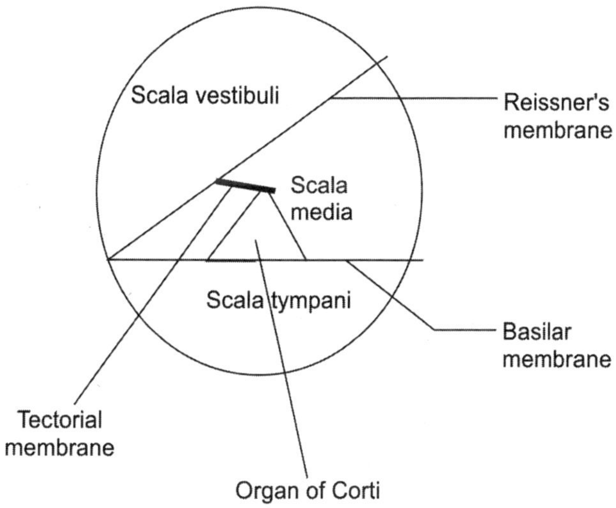

Fig. 12.1: Inner ear

Linear acceleration and gravity: Utricle (horizontal), saccule (vertical)
Angular acceleration: Semicircular canals (crista ampullaris)
Rinne's—NEGATIVE = POSITIVE for conductive deafness

RATIOS

1.3:1	Handle of malleus to process of incus
14:1	TM: Oval window
8:1	Pressure exerted between above two

Wullstein Tympanoplasty

1	Myringoplasty
2	Absent long process of incus
3	Graft placed over stapedial head
4	Graft placed over round window (baffle effect)
5	Fenestration operation of horizontal scc
6	Sinoinversion technique where sound waves are not allowed to hit oval window

Tympanogram Types

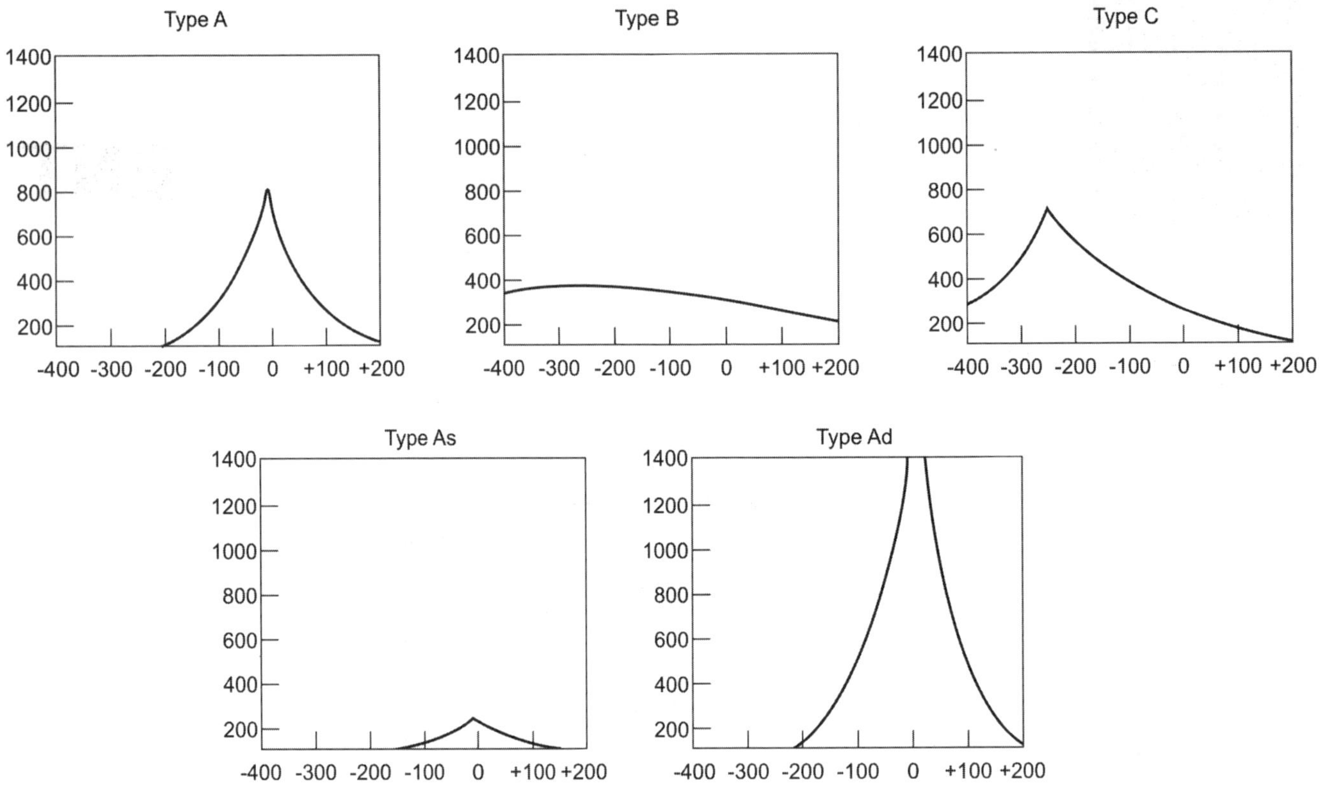

a – Normal, As – otosclerosis, b – fluid in middle ear, Ad – disruption of ossicle, C – retracted TM

Fig. 12.2: Tympanogram

Cochlear deafness	Retrocochlear deafness
Recruitment phenomenon +	Rollover phenomenon +
SISI +	Tone decay + reduced speech discrimination +
Beksey II	Bekesy III

Abscesses

- Bezold: SCM
- Citelle: Posterior belly of digastric
- Lues: Antrum with osseus meatus.

Tobey ayre's sign: Compression of EJV= inc csf pressure
Crowe-becker: No engorgement of retinal veins.

Longitudinal temporal bone #	Transverse temporal bone #
Parallel to EAC	Perpendicular to EAC
CSF otorrhea +	-
Bleeding +	-
Conductive deafness +	SNHL +
Distal 7th N palsy	Proximal 7th nerve palsy

Meniere's Disease

- Male
- Vertigo first, then HOH
- Tullio phenomenon +
- Hennebert's sign
- BERA: Reduced latency of 5th wave
- Lermoyez syndrome: HOH first then vertigo.

Otosclerosis

- Females
- Gelle's test +
- Cahart's notch at 2kHz +
- Schwartz sign +: Flamingo pink TM
- Paracusis of Willisi: Hears well in noisy environment.

Signs in Glomus Tumor

- Brown sign: Blanches the tumor with seiglization
- Aquino sign: Blanching with compression of carotid
- Phelp sign: Erosion of carotico-jugular spine on ct.

Acoustic Neuroma

- Radio resistant, high frequency hearing loss
- Hitzelberger sign: Reduced sensation in posterior metal wall.

Epistaxis Areas

- Brown's area: Posterior aspect, HTN bleed
- Little's area: (anastamosis)
  a. Anterior ethmoid (ICA branch)
  b. Superior labial
  c. Sphenopalatine
  d. Greater palatine (last 3 from ECA)

Woodruff's area: Posterior end of inferior turbinate (sphenopalatine and post pharyngeal).

Retrocolumellar vein: Venous bleed in child.

Cells

- Haller cell: Orbit floor
- Onodi cell: Related to Optic N.
- Aggar nasi: Near the frontal sinus opening.

Cottle's

- Line: through nasal process of frontal bone to maxiallary crest anteriorly.
- Test: pull cheek outward, obstruction is relieved.

Most Commonly Affected Sinuses

- Sinsusitis: M > E > F > S
- Mucocele: F > E > M > S
- In children: Ethmoid

Esophagus landmarks

15 cm	Cricopharynx C6
25 cm	Arch of aorta
28 cm	Tracheal carina
40 cm	LES

Nasal septum #
Chevallet's fracture: Vertical, blow from below
Jarjaway's fracture: Horizontal parallel to blow.

Nasal carcinoma
SCC: NICKEL
Adeno: Ca Wood dust.

Larynx

Abductor	Posterior cricoarytenoid
Adductor	Lateral, transverse and thyroarytenoid and cricothyroid
Tensor	Vocalis (inferior part of thyroarytenoid), cricothyroid
Relaxor	Thyroarytenoid
Opening	Thyroepiglotticus
Closing	Aryepiglotticus

Superior laryngeal nerve		Recurrent laryngeal nerve	
Unilateral	Loss of tension, anesthesia, askew position	**Unilateral**	Paramedian position, improves in 6 months
Bilateral	Breathy voice, aspiration	**Bilateral**	**Stridor +**

Both nerves B/L: CADAVERIC POSITION

Isshiki thyroplasty

I	Medialization of cord, U/L RLN palsy
II	Lateralization
III	AP shortening in puberphonia
IV	AP lengthening in androphonia

TB Larynx Features

- Interarytenoid granulation
- Affects posterior larynx (lupus is anterior)
- Earliest weakness is seen in Adductors
- Mouse nibbled cords
- Turban epiglottis.

Disease Affecting Posterior Larynx

- TB
- GERD
- Intubation granuloma.

LeForte's Fracture

I	Floating palate (Guerin)
II	Floating maxilla
III	**Donkey face**/Craniofacial dissociation

ENT
Larynx

VOCAL CORD

Action	Muscles
Abduction	Posterior cricoarytenoid
Adduction	Thyroarytenoid Lateral cricoarytenoid Cricothyroid
Tensor	Vocalis (internal part of thyroarytenoid) Cricothyroid
Relaxor	Thyroarytenoid
Opening	Thyroepiglotticus
Closing	Aryepiglotticus

NERVE PALSY

Palsy	Defect	Treatment
Unilateral superior laryngeal nerve (SLN) palsy	Loss of tension Anesthesia Askew position	
Bilateral superior laryngeal nerve palsy	Breathy voice Aspiration	
Unilateral adductor palsy (SLN and RLN palsy)	Cadaveric position	
Unilateral recurrent laryngeal nerve palsy	Vocal cord in paramedian position	Type 1 thyroplasty Improves in 6 months
Bilateral recurrent laryngeal nerve palsy	Stridor Voice normal	Tracheostomy Kashima operation

Isshiki Thyroplasty

- Type I – Medialization unilateral rec laryngeal nerve palsy
- Type II – Lateralisation Spasmodic dysphonia
- Type III – Anteroposterior shortening Puberophonia
- Type IV – Anteroposterior lengthening Androphonia.

Lesions Affecting Posterior Larynx

- TB larynx
- Contact pachyderme
- Intubation granuloma
- GERD

TB Larynx

- Earliest: Adductor weakness
- Inter arytenoid granulation
- Posterior larynx involvement
- Mouse nibbed appearance
- Turban epiglottis.

DEEP FASCIA OF NECK

- Prevertebral fascia: Axillary sheath
- Investing layer: Parotid, omohyoid tendon
- Pretracheal fascia: Thyroid, Suspensory ligament of Berry.
- Le Fort fractures of skull involving maxilla:
- Le fort I: Floating palate – Guerin
- Le Fort II: Pyramidal #—Floating maxilla, orbital floor, Infraorbital nerve injury, CSF rhinorrhea
- Le Fort III: Cranio facial dissociation, Donkey face , CSF rhinorrhea

Positions

Boyce position (Barking dog)

- Bronchoscopy
- Esophagoscopy
- Indirect laryngoscopy.

Rose Position

- Thyroidectomy
- Tonsillectomy
- Tracheostomy.

Retropharyngeal Abscess

- Retropharyngeal space (*Gillete space*) : Child > 14 mm
- : Adult > 22 mm
- Node of Henle (Temporary) : Acute retropharyngeal abscess
- Node of Rouvier (Permanent) : Chronic retropharyngeal abscess

Nasal Bone Fracture

- Chavallet #—Vertical—Blow from below
- Jarjavay #—Horizontal—Blow from front
- Correction of septum—Ash forceps
- Correction of nasal bone—Walsham forceps.

ETHMOIDAL SINUS CELLS

- Haller cell: Related to orbital floor
- Onodi cell: Related to optic nerve and internal carotid artery
- Agger nasi cell: Near frontal sinus, anterior most ethmoidal cell.

Meatus

- *Inferior meatus* – Nasolacrimal duct opening
- *Middle meatus* – Frontal, Anterior ethmoidal and Maxillary sinus openings (FAM) from anterior to posterior
- *Superior meatus* – Posterior ethmoidal sinus and sphenoidal sinus opening.

Epistaxis Areas

- Little's area: *(Anterior)* or Kiesselbach's plexus
  - Anterior ethmoidal artery (ophthalmic Art) - *Internal carotid artery*
  - Superior labial artery (facial Art)
  - Sphenopalatine artery (maxillary Art)
  - Greater palatine artery (maxillary Art)

  } *External carotid artery*
- Brown's area: *(posterior)*
  - Hypertensive bleed
- Woodruff's area: *(posterior end of inferior turbinate)*
  - Sphenopalatine artery
  - Posterior pharyngeal artery
- Venous bleed in children: Retrocolumnar vein
- Cottle's line: Line through nasal process of frontal and maxillary bone
- Cottle's area: Vestibular, valvular, attic, turbinal and choanal
- Cottle's test: Pull the cheek outward, vestibular component.

TWO LINERS

- Crooked nose: Tip of the nose in midline
- Deviated nose: Tip of the nose deviated.
- Potts peculiar tumor: Infected sebaceous cyst
- Potts puffy tumor: Osteomyelitis of frontal sinus.
- Darrier's line: Crease on the tip of nose (Allergic rhinitis)
- Dennis Morgan line: Spasm of Muller's muscle.
- Dentigerous cyst: Follicular cyst – unerrupted 3rd molar
- Dental cyst: Radicular cyst – Dental caries, periapical cyst, most common odontogenic cyst.
- Sinusitis: Maxillary → Ethmoidal → Frontal → Sphenoidal (MEFS)
- Mucocoele: Frontal → Ethmoidal → Maxillary → Sphenoidal (FEMS).
- Tobey Ayer test: Compression of external jugular vein (EJV) – increased CSF pressure
- Crow Beck's test: Compression of EJV – no engorgement of retinal and superior ophthalmic veins.
- Arnold nerve: 10th nerve
- Jacobson nerve: 9th nerve.
- Myringotomy: Incision in posteroinferior quadrant
- Grommet: Anteroinferior quadrant.

HEARING LOSS

Cochlear	Retrocochlear
Recruitment	Rollover
SISI positive	Decreased speech discrimination
Bekesy II	Bekesy III

Temporal Bone Fractures

Longitudinal fracture	Transverse fracture
Parallel to external auditory canal	Perpendicular to external auditory canal
CSF otorrhea	-
Bleeding	-
Conductive deafness	Sensory neural deafness
Distal and 7th nerve palsy	Proximal 7th nerve palsy

Wullstein Tympanoplasty

Type	Indication and Procedure
1	Tympanic membrane repair *(Myringoplasty)*
2	Absent long process of malleus
3	Malleus and Incus absent Graft placed over stapes head *(Columella effect)*
4	Only mobile stapes, foot plate present Graft placed in between oval and round window *(Baffle effect)*
5	Opening in lateral (Horizontal) canal *(Fenestration)*
6	Protect oval window, sound waves to round window *(Sinoinversion)*

TYMPANOGRAM

Type	Cause
A	Normal
As	Otoscerosis, Tympanosclerosis and tumor in middle ear
Ad	Disruption of ossicles
B	Fluid in middle ear, tympanic membrane perforation
C	Eustachian tube catarrh, retracted tympanic membrane

FREQUENCIES

Impedence audiometry: 220 Hz
Turning fork : 512 Hz

ENT HEAD MIRROR

- Diameter: 10 cm
- Hole: 19 mm
- Focal length: 25 cm.

Menier's Disease

- Males
- Hard of hearing first followed by vertigo
- Diplacusis

- *Tullio phenomenon*: Noise induced vertigo due to labrynthine fistula
- *Hennebert sign:* False positive fistula test
- Recruitment
- BERA: Decreased latency of V.

Otosclerosis

- Female
- Autosomal dominant
- Hard of hearing for low frequencies first
- As tympanogram
- *Gelle's test:* Test of bone conduction and examines the effect of increased air pressure in the ear canal on hearing using Siegel speculum, no increase in sound
- *Caharts notch:* Dip at 2000 Hz in audiogram
- *Schwartz sign:* Flamingo pink flush of tympanic membrane due to increased vascularity
- *Paracusis willisii:* Good hearing in noisy surrounding
- HRCT is the investigation of choice.

Glomus Tumor

- Female predominant
- Hypotympanum tumor
- Kind of paraganglioma
- Conductive hearing loss
- Pulsatile tinnitus
- Palsy of 9, 10, 11 cranial nerves (Jugular foramen syndrome)
- Ascending pharyngeal and stylomastoid branch of ophthalmic artery embolism
- *Brown sign*: On applying air with Siegel speculum – increased pulsation and blanching
- *Aquino sign*: Blanching on compression of internal carotid artery
- *Phelp sign*: Erosion of corticojugular spine seen in CT.

Acoustic Neuroma (Shwannoma)

- Common cerebello pontine tumor
- Involves 5, 9, 10, 11 cranial nerves
- Trigeminal nerve is the earliest to involve. Absence of corneal sensation is a simple test to check
- High frequency hearing loss
- Radio resistant tumor
- MRI: Gadolinum enhanced is the investigation of choice.

CHAPTER 13

Ophthalmology

Microcornea: < 10 mm

- Fetal alcohol syndrome
- Weil Marchasani syndrome
- Cornellia de Lange
- Turnes syndrome
- Waardenbergh syndrome
- Nance-Horan syndrome.

Megalocornea: > 13 mm

- Marfan's syndrome
- Ehlers-Danlos syndrome
- Osteogenesis imperfecta.

LASERS

Procedure	Laser
Postcapsulotomy Irodotomy Vitreolysis	ND YAG laser
Trabeculoplasty	Argon green
Retinal photocoagulation	Frequency doubled NDYAG, argon green, diode, krypton
PRK LASER LASIK	Excimer Argon, fluoride
Lamellar corneal surgery	Neodymium glass
Laryngeal surgery	CO_2 laser
TURP	Holmium green
Ureteric stone	Holmium yag

Salt and pepper retinopathy causes: Rubella/syphilis (both congenital), LHON, Thioridazine

Sauce and cheese: CMV

Dot and fleck: Alport syndrome

Refractive Index

Aqueous humor	1.336
Vitreous humor	1.36
Cornea	1.376
Lens cortex	1.386
Lens core	1.406

DIMENSIONS

- Macula: 5.5 mm
- Fovea: 1.5 mm
- Foveola: 0.35 mm.

E = A – 2.5L – 0.9K

A – Constant
L – Length
K – Keratometer

Sodium hyaluronate: Viscoelastic + cohesive – shallow AC

Chondritin sulfate: Viscoelastic + dispersive.

Epidemic keratoconjunctivitis	Adenovirus 8, 9
Pharyngoconjunctival fever	Adenovirus 3, 4, 7
Hemorrhagic conjunctivitis	Enterovirus 70

Organisms Penetrating Intact Cornea: Corynebacterium diphtheriae and gonococcus

Pupil	Characters
Argyll Robertson	Accomodation absent, light reflex present
Adie's	Tonic/sluggish/sensitive to pilocarpine/anisocoria +
Marcus-gunn	RAPD/swinging flashlight +
Hutchison	3rd nerve palsy in tentorial herniation
Wernicke's hemianopic pupil	Hemianopic, light reflex absent in the hemianopic field, lesion before LGB

Field of Vision: Blue > Yellow > Red > Green

Optic nerve head	1.5 mm (H) and 1.75 mm (V)
Fovea	1.5 mm
Foveola	.35 mm
Macula	5.5 mm

Vernal KC Features

- Pseudogerontoxon
- Maxwell Lyon sign (ropy discharge)
- Shield ulcer
- Horner Trantas spots.

EMBRYOLOGY OF EYE: DERIVATIVES

Neuroectoderm

- Smooth muscle iris
- Iris and ciliary epithelium
- RPE, retina
- Optic vesicle cup
- Optic nerve.

Surface Ectoderm

- Corneal and conjunctival epithelium
- Lacrimal gland
- Tarsal gland
- Lens.

Mesoderm

- Iris
- Sclera
- Choroid
- Corneal stroma
- Part of vitreous.

Neural Crest

- Corneal endothelium
- Ciliary muscle
- Melanocyte
- Sclera
- Orbital bones
- Ciliary ganglion
- Meningeal sheath of optic nerve
- Orbital connective tissue.

Entropion

Involutional

- Weiss
- Bich modification of Reeh
- Tuckling of inferior rectus.

Cicatricial

- Modified burrow
- Modified kutssey
- Fox procedure.

Spastic

- Botulinum.

Ectropion

Senile, Involutional

- Byron Smith modified Kuhnt
- Bicks.

Cicatricial

- Z plasty.

Paralytic

- Tarsorrhaphy.

Ptosis

- Fasanella sarvat
- Levator resection (conjunctival approach—Blaskowitz) (skin approach—everbusch)
- Frontalis suspension.

Nystagmus

Seesaw	Parachiasmatic
Convergence retraction	Parinaud syndrome
Upbeat nystagmus	Vermis, cerebellum
Downbeat	Arnold Chiari malformation
Gaze evoked	Alcohol, sedatives, cerebellum
Gaze paretic	Pons

Toxic Optic Neuritis

Tobacco

Methanol/ethanol

Cannabis

Lead

Arsenic

CO/CN/CS2

Drugs and ON

Quinidine

Ethambutol/INH

Streptomycin

Digoxin

Amiodarone

Vigabatrin

NSAIDs

Maculopathy and Drugs

Canthaxantin

Thioridazine

Chlorpromazine

Methoxyflurane

Tamoxifen.

Leucocoria

Cong. cataract

RB

ROP

RD

Coat's

Toxocara

Leukemic ophthalmopathy

Causes of Enlarged Corneal Nerves

Cong. glaucoma	Acanthamoeba
Keratoconus	Leprosy
Type 2b MEN	Trauma
Refsum	Fuch's endothelial dystrophy

ROP screening : 31–33 weeks/4–6 weeks post natal/all babies < 28 weeks or < 1500 g

ON GLIOMA : Proptosis first, **ON Meningioma**: Visual impairment first.

CHAPTER 14

General Medicine

Hypovolemic Hyponatremia

- Renal Na loss
- GI Na loss.

Euvolemic Hyponatremia

- Polydipsia
- SIADH
- Hypothyroidism.

Hypervolemic Hyponatremia

- CCF
- CRF
- Cirrhosis
- Nephritic syndrome.

Hypertonic Contraction

Addisons disease, DI.

Isotonic Contraction

- GI-diarrhea
- Renal-Salt losing nephropathy.

Child-Pugh Score

- Bilirubin
- Serum albumin
- PT
- Ascites
- Hepatic encephalopathy.

PELD

- Bilirubin
- Serum, Albumin
- INR
- Age
- Nutrition status.

MELD

- Bilirubin
- Creatinine
- INR.

Renal Colic

- PVJ/Upper ureter: Testis
- Mid ureteric: Mc Burneys
- Lower ureter: Inner side of thigh, groin
- Intramural: Strangury.

Autoantibodies

Antismooth muscle Ab	Autoimmune hepatitis
Antimitochondrial Ab	Primary biliary cirrhosis
Antiendomysial Ab	Celiac sprue
Antisaccharomyces Ab	Crohns disease

Microvascular Steatosis

- Reye syndrome
- Drugs and toxins: Tetracycline, valproic acid
- Acute fatty liver of pregnancy.

Macrovesicular Steatosis

- Alcohol
- Insulin resistance
- Dysbetalipoproteinemia
- Starvation, PEM
- TPN
- Drugs: Aspirin, vitamin A, glucocorticoids, amiodarone
- IBD.

Micronodular Cirrhosis

- Alcohol
- Primary biliary cirrhosis
- Indian childhood cirrhosis
- Hemochromatosis
- Cystic fibrosis
- Bile obstruction
- Intestinal bypass.

Macronodular Cirrhosis

- Chronic viral hepatitis
- Wilsons
- Alpha 1 antitrypsin

- NAFLD
- Hereditary hemorrhagic telangiectasia
- Drugs and toxins

Cholestasis

- CPZ
- Chlorpropamide
- Erythromycin.

Fatty Liver

- Anti HCV
- Tetracycline
- Sodium valproate
- Amiodarone.

Liver Necrosis

- Ccl4
- Phosphorus
- DDT
- Acetaminophen
- Amanita phylloides.

Granuloma Liver

- Phenylbutazone
- Allopurinol
- Sulfonamide
- Quinidine
- Diltiazem
- CBZ.

Autoimmune Hepatitis

- Type I = ANA/SMA abs
- Type 2 = LKM 1 Ab
- Type 3 = Anti-SLA
- LKM 1 = Autoimmune hepatitis
- LKM 2 = Drug-induced hepatitis
- LKM 3 = Chronic hepatitis.

Juvenile Rheumatoid Arthritis

- Pauciarticular <= 4 joints:
- Type 1: ANA positive, RA negative, HLA DR 5/8
- Type 2: ANA negative, RA negative, HLA B 27
- Polyarticular > = 5 joints
- RA positive, ANA positive

Congenital Syphilis

Early-periostitis, bullous, HSM, anemia, thrombocytopenia
Late-interstital keratitis, gumma, 8th nerve deafness, clutton joints.

ST Elevation

- Acute MI
- Prinzmetal angina
- Ventricular aneurysm
- Acute pericarditis
- Early depolarization syndrome
- LVH/LBBB.

Uncommon Causes

- Tako-tsubo syndrome
- Brugada syndrome
- Class Ic antiarrhythmics
- DC conversion
- Myocardial injury
- Hyperkalemia
- Hypercalcemia
- Hypothermia.

Hyperkalemia

- Peaking T wave
- Wide QRS
- Low and wide P wave
- PR prolongation.

Hypokalemia

- ST depression
- Flat/inversion of T wave
- Prominent U wave.

Pericarditis: PR Depression Pathognomonic

Stage 1	ST elevation >=2 leads of V2 to V6, ST depression aVR,V1, PR interval reduced
Stage 2	ST returns to normal
Stage 3	T wave inversion
Stage 4	ECG normalize

Endocarditis

- **MCC of subacute IE:** Strep. viridans
- **MCC of native valve endocarditis:** Staph. aureus
- **MCC of prosthetic valve endocarditis:** < 1 yr- CONS >1 yr- Strep. viridans

Pneumonia

- MCC lobar pneumonia: Strep. pneumonia
- MCC bronchopneumonia: Staph. aureus

Autosomal Dominant Diseases

- Huntington's chorea
- Acute intermittent porphyria
- Factor V leiden mutation
- Familial hypercholesterolemia
- Long QT syndrome
- von Willebrand disease
- Primary pulm. HT
- Neurohypophyseal DI
- MODY
- Familial hypocalciuric hypercalcemia
- MEN
- Hyper IgE recurrent infection syndrome (Job's syndrome)
- C1 esterase deficiency
- Dystrophia myotonica
- Tuberous sclerosis
- Malignant hyperthermia
- Waardenberg syndrome.

Autosomal Recessive

- Albinism
- Alpha 1 antitrypsin deficiency
- Harthup disease
- Hemochromatosis
- Wilsons
- Homocysteinuria
- Glycogen storage disorders
- Galactosemia
- Lysosomal storage disorders
- Cystic fibrosis
- Usher syndrome
- Phenylketonuria
- Sickle cell and thalassemia

- Leukocyte adhesion deficiency
- Chediak-Higashi syndrome
- Fanconis anemia
- Myeloperoxidase deficiency
- Cong. adrenal hyperplasia
- Pendred syndrome
- Friederich ataxia
- Neurogenic muscular atrophy
- Alkaptonuria
- Psteopetrosis
- Klippel feil
- Ehler danlos
- Bartner and Gitelman syndrome
- Nephrogenic DI
- Familial Mediterranean fever
- Bloom syndrome
- Cong. Erythropoietic porphyria
- Acrodermatitis enteropathicae.

X-linked Recessive

- DMD
- Hemophilia
- Color blindness
- Chr. granulomatous disease
- Agammaglobulinemia
- Wiskott Aldrich syndrome
- DI-nephrogenic
- Fragile X syndrome
- Fabry disease
- Menky disease
- Lesch Nyhan syndrome
- G6PD
- Ocular albinism
- Hunter's disease
- Sideroblastic anemia
- Kennedy disease

- Kallman's syndrome
- SCID
- PNH
- OTC deficiency.

X-linked Dominant

- Vitamin D resistant rickets
- Pseudohypoparathyroidism
- Hypophosphatemic rickets
- Incontinentia pigmenta
- Orofaciodigital syndrome
- Rett syndrome
- Aicardi syndrome: Agenesis of corpus callosum
- Goltz syndrome
- Pentalogy of Cantrell.

BROADMANN'S AREAS

Parietal (Sensory)

3,1,2	Primary sensory areas
5,7	Sensory associated areas,stereognosis
39,40	Secondary sensory area, agnosia
43	Taste

Temporal (Psychic)

41,42	Primary auditory
22	Secondary auditory, audiopsychic area
Occipital:	
17	Primary visual
18,19	Visuopsychic

Frontal (Movement and emotion)

4	Primary motor
6,8	Premotor,supplementary motor, frontal eyefield
44,45	Broca's are: motor speech
9,10	Prefrontalemotion, judgement
28	Olfactory bulb

Peripartum Cardiomyopathy

1. 1 month before or 5 months after delivery
2. LV EF < 45%
3. LV EDD: 2.7 cm/metre square.

Nephrotic Syndrome

- Minimal change disease
- FSGS
- MN
- DM
- Amyloidosis
- Fabrys
- Fibrillary immunotactoid disease
- Light chain deposit disease.

AML

Bad Prognostic Factors

- Monosomy 5, 7
- Deletion
- Complete karyotype
- Inversion 3
- FLT3 duplication
- Absence of auer rods
- Preceding MDS
- Extremes of age.

Good Prognosis

- T 8, 21
- T 15, 17
- Inversion 16
- Auer rod
- M 2, 3, 4.

ALL

Good Prognosis

- Female
- Hyperploidy
- 3 to 7 years
- T 12, 21
- L1 type.

NEUROBLASTOMA

Good Prognosis

- < 18 months
- TRK A
- CD 44
- Hyperploidy
- Intramural calcification
- 1, 2, 4s stage.

Lymphatic Mets with Sarcoma

- Angiosarcoma
- Synovial sarcoma
- Epithelial sarcoma
- Clear cell sarcoma
- Lymphosarcoma
- Rhabdomyosarcoma
- Malign. Fibrous histiocytoma.

Papillary Ca Variant

- Follicular
- Diffuse sclerosing
- Tall cell columnar.

Polycythemia Vera

Major Criteria

- Hb > 18.5 in males
- Hb > 16.5 in females
- Jak 2 mutation
- Splenomegaly
- BCR-ABL
- Normal spo2

Minor

- Biopsy
- Decreased erythropoietin levels
- Increased platelets, wbc
- Increased leucocyte alkaline phospatase.

EXTRAHEPATIC MANIFESTATIONS

Hepatitis B

- MN
- PAN
- Arthritis.

Hepatitis C

- MPGN
- DM
- Porphyria
- Sjogrens
- Hypothyroidism
- Cryoglobulinemia.

Metabolic Acidosis

High Anion Gap (Anion excess)

- DKA
- Lactic acidosis
- Starvation
- Renal failure
- Cholera
- Ethylene glycol
- Methanol
- Salicylates
- Pyroglutamic acid.

Low Anion Gap or Hyperchloremic

- RTA
- CA inhibitors
- Diarrhea
- Ingesting ammonium chloride
- Pancreatic damage
- Multiple myeloma.

Low C3

- MPGN, PIGN
- SLE
- Cryoglobulinemia
- Shunt nephritis
- Liver disease
- Pancreatitis
- Felty syndrome.

Normal C3

- IgA
- HUS
- Anti GBM
- Vasculitis
- Pauciimmune
- Fibrillary nephropathy
- Vasculitis.

RPGN/Crescentric

Type 1 (Anti GBM)

- Idiopathic
- Goodpasture's syndrome.

Type 2 (Immune complex)

- Idiopathic
- PIGN

- SLE
- MPGN
- Henoch sconlein purpura
- IgA.

Type 3 (Pauci immune)

- Idiopathic
- Wegener's
- Churg-Strauss
- Microscopic polyangiopathy.

Type 4: ANCA+, GBM+

Type 5: ANCA Negative, Pauciimmune

Channelopathies:

Potassium

- Episodic ataxia
- Benign neonatal familial convulsion
- Jervell and Lange-Nielsen syndrome—long QT
- Autosomal dominant progressive deafness.

Calcium

- Episodic ataxia 2
- Spinocerebellar ataxia
- Familial hemiplegic migraine
- Hypokalemic periodic paralysis.

Sodium

- Generalized epilepsy with febrile convulsions
- Hyperkalemic periodic paralysis
- Myotonia congenital.

Chloride

- Myotonia congenital.

Deposits

Subepithelial	PSGN, RPGN
Subendothelial	MPGN 1, SLE
Epimembranous	MN, Hegmann
Intramembranous	MPGN 2
Mesangial	IgA, HSP

Lynch Syndrome (HNPCC)

- Ca endometrium
- Ca colon
- Ca ovary

- Ca bileduct
- Ca small intestine
- Ca stomach
- Ca pancreas
- Ca renal pelvis
- Ca ureter
- Ca bladder
- Skin cancer
- Except liver and renal parenchyma.

Massive Splenomegaly

- CML
- CLL
- Hairy cell leukemia
- Lymphoma
- Myelofibrosis
- Polycythemia vera
- Autoimmune hemolytic anemia
- Diffuse splenic hemangioma
- Gauchers disease
- Sarcoidosis.

Papillary Necrosis

(POSTCARD)

- Pyelonepritis
- Obstruction
- Sickle cell disease
- TB
- Cirrhosis
- Analgesic abuse
- Renal vein thrombosis
- Diabetes.

Plasmapheresis

- Anti-GBM, RPGN
- Refsums disease
- Myasthenia gravis, Lambert-Eaton
- AIDP CIDP
- TTP
- Post transfusion purpura
- Myeloma
- MS
- Cryoglobulinemia
- Sydenham's chorea.

Pseudomembranous Enterocolitis

Cl. difficile, clindamycin causes it.

Treatment

- Metronidazole
- Vancomycin/teicoplanin
- Bacitracin/fusidic acid.

Descending Paralysis

- Polio
- Tetanus
- Botulinism
- Diphtheria.

Hemoperfusion

- Chloramphenicol
- Disopyramide
- Procainamide
- Phenol
- Theophylline
- Sedatives.

Type 1 RTA

- Distal
- Decreased H ions
- Hypokalemia
- Increased urine Ca
- Positive anion gap
- Decreased urine citrate
- Stones
- Urine pH > 5.5.

Type 2 RTA

- Proximal
- Fanconi syndrome
- Increased bicarbonate loss
- Increased urine calcium
- Severe hypokalemia
- Increased urine citrate.

Trinucleotide Repeat

- Huntingtons disease (CAG)
- Spinocerebellar ataxia (1.2.3.6.7.17) CAG (8.12) CTG
- Spinomuscular atrophy
- Dentatorubraopallidosylvian atrophy (CAG)
- Friederich ataxia (GAA)

- Fragile X syndrome (CGG)
- Myotonic dystrophy (CTG).
  - Negative anion gap
  - No stones
  - Urine pH < 5.5.

Type 3

Mixed.

Type 5

- Hyperkalemia
- Hypoaldosteronism.

Anemia

- Serum ferritin decreased only in iron deficiency anemia.
- Serum ferritin is increased in anemia of chronic disease.
- TIBC normal or decreased in anemia of chronic disease and sideroblastic anemia.
- Serum iron and transferring saturation decreased in iron def. anemia and anemia of chronic disease
- TIBC-normal in thalassemia
- Microcytosis preced hypochromia in iron def.anemia
- Free erythroporphyrin increased in iron def. anemia and anemia of chronic disease.

		Iron-deficiency anemia	Thalasemia
Mentzer index	MCV/RBC	> 13	< 13
RDW index	(MCV× RDW)/RBC	> 220	< 220
RDW		> 13	normal

Transferring saturation = (serum iron/TIBC) × 100

Mitochondrial Disorders

1. PEARSON (PEAR) syndrome: Pancreas and bone marrow failure
2. NARP: Neurogenic ataxia RP
3. LHON: Lobers hereditary optic neuropathy
4. MELAS: Mitochondrial myopathy encephalopathy lactic acidosis stroke
5. MERRF: Mitochondrial myopathy epilepsy red ragged fibre disease
6. MMC: Mitomyopathy with cardiomyopathy
7. ADMIMY: Autosomal dominant mitochondrial inherited myopathy
8. Leig: Progressive neurologic with basal ganglia, increased lactate in CSF
9. Kearn-Sayre syndrome: Ophthalmoplegia, RP, cardiomyopathy, complete heart block
10. CPEO: Congenital progressive ophthalmoplegia.

DNA Repair Disease

Xeroderma pigmentosum	Nucleotide excision repair
Ataxia telangiectasia	
Fanconis anemia	Defective repair of cross linkage
Bloom syndrome	DNA ligase
HNPCC	Mismatch repair, microsatellite instability

Meningitis

Neonates	E. coli, group B streptococcus, Chromobacter Meningosepticum, Listeria
2 months to 2 years	Hemophilus influenza B
> 2 years	Pneumococcus (deafness)
Anytime	Meningococcus

Vaccines

OPV: Freeze, $Mgcl_2$

BCG: Normal saline

MMR: Eomycin

Measles: Sc/im, TSST, kanamycin, HIV safe

DPT: Thiomerase, CP not contraindicated, never freeze

6 weeks,10 and 14 weeks: **Hib, Hep B, DPT, Pneumococcus, IPV and OPV**

HPV: Gardasil- Quadrivalent 10 to 26 years (6, 11, 16, 18)

Cervarix: Bivalent 10 to 45 years (16, 18, 31, 35)

Varicella: > 1 year

Hep A: > 2 years – 0, 6

Meningococcus: > 2 years

Typhoid: Vi > 2 years, oral > 6 years booster every 3 years.

EEG

Absence seizures: 3 hz generalized spike and wave pattern, sudden onset and offset

Prion disease: CJD-scattered Q activity, stereotyped periodic bursts, repetitive high voltage triphasic and polyphasic in advanced cases

SSPE: Periodic high voltage, sharp S low waves, followed by attenuated background, *burst suppression*

Viral encephalitis: Periodic focal temporal lobe background of slow and attenuated

Encephalitis/acute stroke: PLEDS, periodic lateralized epileptiform discharge

Juvenile myotonic epilepsy: Bursts 4–6 hz irregular polyspike

Hepatic encephalopathy: Stage 1, 2, 3- triphasic; stage 4-s waves(delta)

Schizophrenia: Decreased alpha activity

Alzheimers disease: Diffuse slow wave in delta range 4 to 7 hz

Tall Stature

- Cerebral gigantism
- Homocysteinuria
- Weaver syndrome
- Fragile X
- Marfans syndrome
- Kleinfelters syndrome
- Beckwith Wiedmann syndrome.

Constitutional

- Bone < chronological age
- Bone age = height age.

Familial

- Bone age = chronological age
- Bone age > height age.

Brain Tumors

< 1 year	Supratentorial (choroid plexus, teratoma)
1 to 10 years	Infratentorial (juvenile piloastrocytic, medulloblastoma)
> 10 years	Supratentorial (astrocytoma)

CCF

- < 3 days : Atresia
- 1 week : TGA, hypoplastic left heart
- 1 to 4 weeks : Coarctation of aorta, TGA
- 1 to 2 months : TAPVC, ALCAPPA, ECD
- > 2 months : AS, VSD, PDA.

Monoclonal Antibodies

MAB	Target	Use
Abciximab	Gp 2b 3a	Antiplatelets
Adalimumab	THF alpha	RA, psoriatic arthropathy
Infliximab	TNF alpha	Crohns, RA
Golimumab	TNF alpha	Crohns, RA
Certolizumab	TNF alpha and T cell	Crohns
Tositumumab	CD 20	B cell NHL
Ibritumomab	CD 20	B cell NHL
Rituximab	CD 20	B cell NHL, RA, EBV
Ocrelizumab	CD 20	SLE
Ofutumumab	CD 20	SLE, CLL, NHL
Alemtuzumab	CD 52	CLL, ALL
Belimumab	BLY8	SLE
Eprutuzumab	CD 22	SLE

Contd...

Contd...

MAB	Target	Use
Tocilizumab	IL 6R	SLE
Efalizumab	CD 11a, LFA	Psoriasis
Ustekinumab	IL 12 , 23	Psoriasis, MS
Talizumab	IgE	Peanut allergy
Omalizumab	IgE	Bronchial asthma
Mepolizumab	IL 5	BA, Eosinophilic esophagitis
Canakinumab	IL 1B	CAPS, RA
Muromonab	CD 3	Immunosuppressant
Daclizumab	IL 2R, CD 25	Immunosuppressant
Basiliximab	IL 2R	Immunosuppressant
Ipilimumab	MDX 101	Advanced melanoma
Bevacizumab	VEGF	Macular gegeneration, colon Ca
Ranibizumab	VEGF	Ca breast, lung, anal canal
Cetuximab	EGFR	Ca colon, head and neck
Panitumumab	EGFR	Ca colon
Nimotuzumab	EGFR	Squamous cell ca, astrocytoma, glioma
Natalizumab	Integrin alpha beta 4	Multiple sclerosis and crohns
Gemtuzumab, ozakamycin	CD 33	AML
Donesumab	RANKL	Osteoporosis
Ecromeximab		Malignant melanoma
Palivizumab	RSV	
Panobacumab	Pseudomonas	
Efungumab	Fungus	Invasive candidiasis
Nacolomab, endrocolomab		Ca colon
Salonezumab	Neuron	Alzheimer's disease
Stamulumab	muscle	Muscular dystrophy
Oregovomab	CA 125	Ovarian tumor
Trastuzumab, pentazumab	Her 2 neu	Breast Ca
Lapatinib	HER 2	Breast Ca
Imatinib	Tyrosine kinase inhibitor	CML, GIST
Nilotinib	Tyrosine kinase inhibitor	CML
Soratinib	Tyrosine kinase inhibitor and VEGFR	RCC, hepatic Ca
Sunitinib	Tyrosine kinase inhibitor, VEGFR, PDGFR	RCC, GIST
Pazopanib	VEGFR, PDGFR	RCC
Erlotinib	Inhibitor RTK PO4	Non small cell Ca lung
Gefnitinib	EGFR	Non small cell Ca lung
pegtinib	Anti VEGF	Macular degeneration
Bortezomin+ lenalidomide	NFK B inhibit, proteasome	Multiple myeloma
Etanercept	TNF alpha	RA
Abatacept	CD 80, 96, costimulator	RA

Contd...

Contd...

MAB	Target	Use
Alefacept	LFA 3	Psoriasis
Rilonacept	IL 1 inhibitors	CAPS Cyroprin associated periodic syndrome
Aldesleukin	Recombinant IL2	Malignant melanoma, RCC
Romidespin, Vorinostat	Histone, deacetylase inhibitor	Cutaneous T cell lymphoma
Anakinra	IL 1 inhibitor	Septic shock RA
Denlileukin deffitox	IL 2, diphtheria toxin	Cutaneous T cell lymphoma
Bexarotene	Retinoid	Cutaneous T cell lymphoma

Monoclonal Antibodies – Concepts

Naming

- *mo* : M omab—murine
- *xi* : Ximab—chimeric
- *u* : Umab—humanised

Target

- **tu** : Tumor
- **li** : Immunity
- **ci** : Circulation
- **vi** : Infection
- **os** : Osteoporosis.

- beta 2 microglobulin: Multiple myeloma
- beta 2 transferrin: CSF rhinnorhea.

HETEROPHILE NEGATIVE INFECTIOUS MONONUCLEOSIS

1. CMV
2. Toxoplasmosis
3. Listeria.

Escape mutant: HBeAg positive

HBsAg negative

Precore mutant: HBeAg negative

Anti-HBeAg positive

Anti-HBSAg positive.

Exercise	Murmur	Mechanism
Squatting	Decrease in MVP & HOCM	Increase in venous return, Increase in endiastolic LV size
Straining phase of valsalva	Increase in MVP & HOCM	Decrease in venous return
Hand grip	Increase in MR & VSD	Increase in afterload

AUTOANTIBODIES

Antibody	Disease
ANA	SLE Sjogrens syndrome Systemic sclerosis Autoimmune hepatitis Mixed connective tissue disorder (MCTD) Dermatomyositis, Polymyositis
Anti ds DNA	SLE – specific
Anti Sm (Smith)	SLE – most specific
Anti histone	Drug induced lupus
Anti- ribosomal P protein	CNS lupus
Anti smooth muscle	Autoimmune hepatitis
Anti U1 - RNP	Mixed connective tissue disorder (MCTD)
Anti – DNA topoisomerase -1 (Scl 70)	Systemic sclerosis
Anti centromere	CREST syndrome (limited scleroderma)
Anti PM / Scl	Scleroderma
Anti histidyl – RNA synthetase	Dermatomyositis, Polymyositis
Anti RO(SS-A) Anti LA (SS-B)	Sjogren syndrome
Anti JO	Polymyositis
Anti Sp100 Anti p62 Anti gp210	Primary biliary cirrhosis
Anti mitochondrial	Primary biliary cirrhosis
Anti GM-1	Traveler's diarrhea
Anti GD3	Guillian Barre syndrome (GBS)
Anti GQ1B	Miller Fisher variant of GBS
Anti aquaporin – 4	Neuromyelitis optica
Anti actin Anti endomysial Anti tissue transglutaminase Anti gliadin	Coeliac disease
Anti saccharomyces (ASCA)	Crohn's disease

CHAPTER 15

Surgery

Named Procedues

Andersen and Hynes	PUJ obstruction
Nesbit	Peyronie's disease
Rovsing	ADPKD
Bentall	Dilated aortic root
Dennis brown	Orchidopexy by narrowing scrotal neck
Burch	Stress incontinence
Boari	Bladder wall fashioned for ureter
Palma	Femoral vein occlusion
Paloma	Varicocele
Dunhill	Near total thyroidectomy
Sistruk	TG cyst
Dowling	Hydatid cyst
Dohlmann	Zenker's diverticulum
Delorome	Rectal prolapse
Frey	Chronic pancreatitis
Duhamel	Pull through operation in Hirschprung
Swenson	Endroectal pull through in Hirsch.
Soave	Coloanal anast. in Hirsch.
Kasai	Biliary atresia
Bishop koop	Meconium ileus
Noble's plication	Recurrent intestinal obstruction
Paul mikulicz	Sigmoid volvulus with impending gangrene
Ramsted	Pyloric stenosis
Heller	Achalasia
Liley	Choledochal cyst
Matthews/Snodgraes	Hypospadias
Millard	Cleft lip

TEF Types

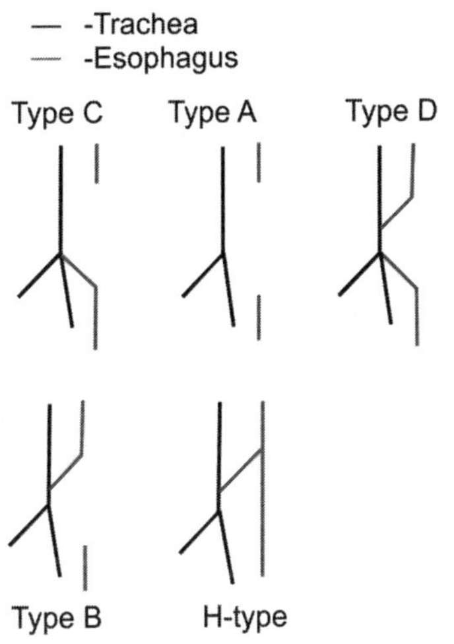

Fig. 15.1: Please provide caption

Bladder Outlet Obstruction

- Flow rate < 10 ml/s
- Pressure > 80 cm H 20
- Residual volume > 150 ml

MC Symptoms in Urology

Wilms'	Mass
RCC	Hematuria
Bladder Ca	Painless hematuria
Bladder stone	Terminal hematuria
TB	Increased frequency
Calculus	Pain
BPH	Increased frequency

Prostate

- Screening for Ca : DRE + PSA
- Diagnosis : PSA + TRUS biopsy
- Staging : CT/MRI

PSA

- < 4 ng/ml : normal
- 4–10 : BPH
- > 10 : Carcinoma
- Gleason : Grade 1–5, score 2–10

Indications for Thoracotomy

- Tracheobronchial ring
- Esophageal/diaphragm rupture
- Cardiac tamponade
- Massive hemothorax
- Major thoracic vessel injury.

MC cause of pancoast tumour is SCC.

MC Mediastinal Masses

- Anterior : Thymus
- Middle : Cyst
- Posterior : Neurogenic

Pseudocyst Surgery (Rule of 6)

- > 6 weeks
- > 6 cm
- > 6 mm thickness.

Zollinger-Ellison Syndrome

NOT ZES if pH > 3

- BAO > 15 m Eq/hr
- Fasting gastrin > 1000 pg/ml
- Tests: Secretin stimulation, calcium infusion, standard meal test
- Imaging: Somatostatin scintigraphy.

Appendiceal Carcinoid

- < 1 cm appendectomy
- 1–2 cm without lymphnode- appendectomy
- 1–2 cm with LN or > 2 cm Rt. Hemicolectomy.

Solitary Rectal Ulcer

- Its due to local ischemia
- M = F
- 20 – 40 years
- **Hypocellular lamina propria with fibrosis**
- **Rx-rectopexy.**

Cholecystectomy Indications

- > 3 cm stone
- Polyp
- Diabetic
- Mucocele
- Porcelain GB
- Post-transplant/immunocompromised.

STAGING OF TUMORS

Breast

- **T1 : Tumor < 2 cm**
- **T2 : Tumor 2–5 cm**
- **T3 : > 5 cm**
- **T4** : T4a – The tumor has spread into the chest wall
- **T4b** : The tumor has spread into the skin
- T4c : The tumor is fixed to both the skin and the chest wall
- T4d : Inflammatory carcinoma.

- **N1 : Mobile axillary LN**
- **N2a : Fixed axillary**
- **N2b : Internal mammary LN**
- **N3a : Infraclavicular**
- **N3b : Internal mammary + axillary**
- **N3c : Supraclavicular.**

Bladder

- **T1 : Mucosa**
- **T2 : Muscular**
- **T3 : Palpable**
- **T4a : Pelvic wall**
- **T4b : Prostate.**

Prostate

- **T1 : Incidental in prostatectomy**
- **T2a : One lobe b: 2 lobes**
- **T3 : Capsule**
- **T4 : Adjacent organs.**

Testis

- **IA : Only testis**
- **IB : Vascular/lymphatic invasion**
- **II : A - node < 2 cm (radio + chemo + Orchidectomy with RPLND)**
  B - node 2–5 cm (radio + chemo + Orchidectomy with RPLND)
  C - node > 5 cm (chemo)
- **III : Metastasis (chemo).**

CHAPTER 16

Obstetrics and Gynecology

Triple Test: Down's Syndrome

- AFP: Reduced
- Estradiol: Reduced
- hCG: High
- Inhibin: High.

Ponderal Index

- >2 = Symmetric IUGR
- <2 = Asymmetric IUGR

Theories of Endometriosis

- Sampson: Retrograde spread
- Meyer and Iwanoff: Coelomic metaplasia
- Halbans: Metastatic.

Pregnancy Signs

- Jacquimer/Chadwick : Bluish anterior vagina
- Osiander : Pulsations in lateral fornix
- Hartman : Implantation bleed
- Goodell : Softening of cervix
- Hegar : Bimanual palpation, soft isthmus
- Palmer : Contraction
- Piskacek sign : One half firm than other.

CERVICAL LENGTH

Time	Cervix : Body
Before puberty	2:1
At puberty	1:2
Reproductive age	1:4

3-SWAB METHYLENE BLUE TEST

Swab-stained	Fistula
Upper	Uretero – Vaginal
Middle	Vescico – Vaginal
Lower	Urethro – Vaginal

Risk of Malignancy in Mole

- > 40 years
- Hcg > 1 lakhs
- Leutin cyst > 6 cm
- H/o mole
- Uterine size > 20 weeks.

Progesterone

- Increased temperature
- Increases weight
- Increases lipids
- Increases thrombus formation.

Estrogen

- Increases fibrinogen
- Increases HDL, increases TGL
- Sodium and water retention
- Closure of epiphysis
- Glycogen deposition.

CELL DIVISION

Day	Chorionicity
4 – 8	Monochorionic diamniotic
8 – 12	Monochorionic monoamniotic
> 13	Conjoined twin

Contraindications of IUCD

- Pregnancy
- PID
- DUB
- Ectopics
- Ca cervix.

Contraindications of OCP

- Pregnancy
- DUB
- Smoker > 35 years
- HT
- Thromboembolism
- Decreased liver function.

PCOD

Increased	Decreased
Estrogen (E2) Androgen LH Prolactin Inhibin LDL TGI	Progesterone FSH Sex hormone binding protein HDL Apo A-1

Named Surgeries

Tubectomy

Pomeroy	0.4% failure
Uchida	Serosa left, broad ligament
Madlener	Crushing
Irwing	Buried in myometrium
Aldrige	Fimbria buried in broad ligament
Clip	2 to 3% failure

Prolapse

Purandhare	Abd. cervicopexy
Kanna, Shirodkar	ASIS sling
Fothergills/Manchester	Amputation of cervix
Kelleys suture	Cystocoel, stress incontinence
Mosckowitz repair	Enterocoel
Fentons	Vaginismus
McIndoe	Vaginal atresia
Strassmann	Bicornuate uterus

Stress Incontinence

Pacey, Kelly	Vaginal
Marshall, Bruch	Abdominal
Pereyra	Combined

Retroversion = Never congenital

- Modified Gilliams
- Baldy Webster
- Plication of round ligament
- Hodge pessary.

Endometrial Thickness

- Not > 4 mm = postmenopausal
- Not > 10 mm = perimenopausal

Decreases in Pregnancy

- Hb
- Factor 11, 13
- Renal: Urea, creatinine, BUN
- Electrolytes
- Albumin
- PVR, DBP
- Platelets.

PLACENTA—ABNORMAL TYPES

Placenta accreta	Adherent placenta to myometrium
Placenta increta	Invades myometrium
Placenta percreta	Penetrates serosa

Diameters

Suboccipitobregmatic	9.5
Suboccipitofrontal	10
Occipitofrontal	11.5
Mentovertical	14
Submentovertical	11.5
Submentobregmatic	9.5
Interspinous diameter	10
Intertuberous diameter	11
Post sagittal diameter	7.5
Bi mastoid	7.5
Bi temporal	8
Bi parietal	9.5
Supersubparietal	8.5
Diagonal conjugate	12
Obstretic diameter	10
True conjugate	11

Asynclitism

Naegele's: Anterior

Litzmann: Posterior.

Pelvis

Naegele's pelvis : One sacral ala absent

Robert's pelvis : Both ala absent

Direct OP : Anthropoid - face to pubis

Persistent OP : Android - deep transverse arrest.

Shoulder Dystocia

Head to shoulder > 1 hour

Maneuvre:

- **McRoberts** : Leg over abdomen
- **Wood's** : Corkscrew post. shoulder first delivery
- **Rubens** : Adduction of shoulder, decreases shoulder to shoulder diameter
- **Zavanelli** : Head OA pushed cesarean.

Forceps

- **Wriggley** : Outlet
- **Killiand** : Deep transverse arrest, asynclitism
- **Piper** : Aftercoming head
- **Das** : Long curved
- **Anderson and Simpson** : Midcavity.

Trial Labor: Contraindications

- Midpelvis/outlet contraction
- Elderly primi
- Previous cesarean
- Malpresentation
- Preeclampsia
- Post maturity
- DM
- Heart disease
- Tuberculosis.

Delivery Not Possible

- Mentoposterior
- Brow
- Transverse lie.

Birth by Flexion

- Persistent OP
- Face.

Only Cesarean

- Placenta previa 2b, 3, 4
- First twin non vertex
- Coarctation of aorta
- Brow
- Monoamniotic monochorionic
- Previous classical
- Twin with previous cesarean
- Persistent mentoposterior.

Classical

- Ca cervix
- High repair VVF
- Lower segment fibroid
- Placenta accrete
- Dense adhesion.

Vaginal Epithelium

- Basal: Extremes of age, postpartum
- Intermediate: Birth, pregnancy, menopause
- Superficial: Reproductive period
  - OCP does not increase breast Ca
  - LNG IUCD decreases PID
  - PID least common with condom
  - Detrusor instability: > 7 times in morning and greater than 1 in night
  - IUCD: 6 weeks normal, 3 months LSCS
  - Fibroid-sarcoma – 0.5%
  - Uterine rupture: LSCS = 0.2–1.5%
  - Classical = 1–7%
  - LSCS with obstruction: Lower segmental rupture
  - Desogestrol: Decreases ovulation
  - DMPA: In sickle cell
  - Ca 125 except PCOD
  - Ca in situ: Vaginal delivery
  - DPCC, phospatidyl glycerol: Blood
  - BRCA 2: Male breast ca

- Tamoxifen: First trimester abortion with mifepristone
- Clomiphene citrate: 2nd day
- IUD: No ARM
- Primaquine: Contraindicated in pregnancy
- Vault ca: 1%.

Weeks	Events	Procedures
0		
2		
4	Gestational sac seen by TVS	
6	Gestational sac seen by TAS and FH by TVS	
8	FH by TAS and max hCG levels	
10	Anencephaly by USG	CVS sampling, sex determination
12	Upto 12 weeks, heparin, afterwards warfarin, suction evacuation upto 12 weeks, urine formation in fetus, breathing and swallowing and insulin secretion commences	
14	Start zidovudine	Amniocentesis, circlage
16	Quickening	
18	Cordocentesis, FH by steth, 16–18 weeks—MSAFP, triple test	
20	Anomaly scan	
22		
24	GTT, no NSAIDs after 24 weeks	
26		
28	Roll over test, surfactant release	
30	Can start parenteral iron	
32	Cardiac output is maximum in mother	
34	< 34 weeks, premature	
36	> restart heparin, stop 6 hours prior to delivery	
37	> 37 weeks, term. terminate in mild PIH	
42	Post term	
2w PP	Uterus is a pelvic organ	
6w PP	Uterus is normal size, end of puerperium	

Gynec. oncology

Ovarian Tumors

Epithelial

- Serous cystenoma: MC malignancy, Fallopian tube, bilateral, pregnancy and psammoma bodies
- Mucinous: Cercix, large tumor, occurs along with dermoid and Brenner tumor, pseudomyxoma peritoni
- Endometroid: Endocervical gland
- Clear cell: Mesonephroid, endometrial and clear cell variant, resemble RCC, Hobnail cell
- Brenner: Transitional epithelium, occurs along with mucinous and dermoid tumor, Walthard cell rest
- Cysadenofibraoma.

Sexcord stromal tumors

- Thecoma: Estrogen secretion, Oil "o" red—positive
- Fibroma: Pseudomeigs syndrome, Oil "o" – negative
- Granulosa cell: Carl Exner bodies, estrogen and inhibin secretion, precocious puberty, mets to opposite ovary
- Sertoli cell: Arrhenoblastoma, androgen secretion (Androblastoma), malignant, raised inhibin
- Hilus cell: Pure leydig cell tumor, androgen secreting, Renke cell, benign tumor
- Small cell
- Gynandroblastoma.

Germ cell tumors

- Teratoma: MC benign ovarian tumor, prone for torsion, occurs in pregnancy, AFP+, hCG–
- Dysgerminoma: Bilateral, AFP–, PLAP+, LDH+, hCG +
- Yolk sac: Endodermal sinus tumor – Schiller Duval bodies, always unilateral, AFP+, m a1 antitripsin +, hCG –
- Choriocarcinoma: Pure is rare, chemo resistant
- Polyembryoma: Embryoid bodies
- Gonadoblastoma: Abnormal sexual development
- Embryonal carcinoma: Highly malignant, AFP+, hCG+, can occur bilaterally.

KRUKENBERG TUMORS

Bilateral waxy smooth surface, no adhesion, shape maintained and signet cells.

- Stomach: MC
- Colon
- Appendix
- Breast (Invasive lobular).

PSEUDO-MEIG'S SYNDROME

- Brenner tumor
- Granulose cell tumor
- Thecoma
- Pedunculated fibroid.

PSEUDO-MYXOMA PERITONEI

- Mucinous carcinoma of ovary
- Appendicular carcinoma
- Mucocele of appendix.

T1a	IA	One ovary, capsule intact
T1b	IB	Both ovaries, capsule intact
T1c	IC	Capsule ruptured, malignant cells in ascites or peritoneal washings
T2a	IIA	Uterus, tube(s)
T2b	IIB	Other pelvic tissues
T2c	IIC	Malignant cells in ascites or peritoneal washings

Contd...

Contd...

T3a	IIIA	Microscopic peritoneal metastasis
T3b	IIIB	Macroscopic peritoneal metastasis <=2 cm
T3c	IIIC	Peritoneal metastasis > 2 cm and/or
N1	IIIC	Regional lymph node metastasis (with any T)
M1	IV	Distant metastasis (excluding peritoneal metastasis)

CA CERVIX STAGING

Tis	0	In situ
T1	I	Confined to uterus
T1a	IA	Diagnosed only by microscopy
T1a1	IA1	Depth = < 3 mm, horizontal spread = < 7 mm
T1a2	IA2	Depth > 3 to 5 mm, horizontal spread = < 7 mm
T1b	IB	Clinically visible or microscopic lesion, greater than T1a2
T1b1	IB1	= < 4 cm
T1b2	IB2	> 4 cm
T2	II	Beyond uterus but not pelvic wall or lower third of vagina
T2a	IIA	No parametrial involvement
T2b	IIB	Parametrial involvement
T3	III	Lower third of vagina or pelvic wall or hydronephrosis
T3a	IIIA	Lower third of vagina
T3b	IIIB	Pelvic wall/hydronephrosis
T4	IVA	Mucosa of bladder or rectum; beyond true pelvis
M1	IVB	Distant metastasis

Curative surgery only upto stage 2a.

CA ENDOMETRIUM

Tis	0	In situ
T1	I	Confined to corpus
T1a	IA	Limited to endometrium
T1b	IB	= < half of myometrium
T1c	IC	> half of myometrium
T2a	IIA	Endocervical glandular only
T2b	IIB	Cervical stroma
T3a	IIIA	Serosa/adnexa/positive peritoneal cytology
T3b	IIIB	Vaginal involvement
T1/2/3-N1	IIIC	Regional lymphnode metastasis
T4	IVA	Mucosa of bladder or bowel
M1	IVB	Distant metastasis

- **Stage Ia and b: TAH with BSO**
- **Stage Ic: 2b – TAH with BSO with RT**
- **>III: No surgery, only RT with chemo.**

Modified WHO Prognostic Scoring System as Adapted by FIGO 2010				
Scores	**0**	**1**	**2**	**4**
Age (years)	< 40	≥ 40	–	–
Antecedent pregnancy	Mole	Abortion	Term	–
Interval in months from end of index pregnancy to treatment	< 4	4 – <7	7 – <13	≥ 13
Pretreatment serum hCG (IU/L)	< 10^3	10^3 – < 10^4	10^4 – < 10^5	> 10^5
Largest tumor size (including uterus)	< 3	3 – < 5 cm	≥ 5 cm	–
Site of metastases	Lung	Spleen, kidney	Gastrointestinal	Liver, brain
Number of metastases	–	1 – 4	5 – 8	> 8
Previous failed chemotherapy	–	–	Single drug	≥ 2 drugs

Modified WHO Prognostic Scoring System as Adapted by FIGO				
Parameters	**Score**			
	0	**1**	**2**	**3**
Age (years)	< 39	> 39	–	–
Antecedent pregnancy	Mole	Abortion	Term	–
Interval in months from end of index pregnancy to treatment (months)	< 4	4 – 6	7 – 12	> 12
Pretreatment serum hCG (IU/L)	10^3	10^3 – 10^4	10^4 – 10^5	> 10^5
ABO group (female X male)		O & A	A & AB	
Largest tumor size (cm)	< 3	3 – 5 cm	> 5 cm	–
Site of metastases		Spleen, kidney	Gastrointestinal, liver	Brain
Number of metastases	–	1 – 4	4 – 8	> 8
Prior chemotherapy	–	–	Single drug	≥ 2 drugs
Total score	< 5	Low risk, 5 – 7	Medium risk, > 7	High risk

Cells	Tumors
Call exner bodies	Granulosa cell tumor
Schiller duval bodies	Endodermal sinus (yolk sac) tumors
Walthard cell nest/puffed wheat	Brenner cell tumor
Signet ring	Krukenberg tumor
Reinle crystal	Hilus cell
Hobnail	Clear cell ca
Rokitanski body	Toratoma
Tennis rachet	Sarcoma botyroides

CHAPTER 17

Pediatrics

PRETERM MILK

Rich in FEPSI-Z   Poor(less) in $CaPO_4$ and lactose

F - Fat
E - Energy
P - Protein
S - Sodium
I - Iron
Z - Zinc

< 30 weeks IV fluids
→ 10% Dextrose, < 3 days
→ N/5 Saline and 10% Dextrose, > 3 days

HR < 60
Chest amp: 90/30 total 120
Moro reflex: Appears at 7th month of IUL (28 to 32 weeks of gestation)—3 m
Disappears at 3rd month of life.

LPS: Not at Birth
STNR (Symmeric Tonic Neck Reflex): Quadruped crawling (cat reflex).

HIE (Hypoxic Ischemic Encephalopathy)

Stage I – Strong moro reflex + Mydriasis
Stage II – Week moro reflex + Miosis
Stage III – Abesnt/ NO moro reflex + unequal pupil

Jaundice (Kramer's Zone)

5 – Head
10 – Umbilicus
12 – Thigh
15 – Legs
> 15 – Palm and soles

Pathological Jaundice

Total Bilirubin (TBR) > 15 mg%
Direct Bilirubin > 2 mg%
↑ 0.5 mg%/hour or ↑ 5 mg%/24 hours
Appearing 1st 24 hours

IUGR

LBW – < 2.5 kg
VLBW – < 1.5 kg
ELBW – < 1 kg

Breastfeeding jaundice : 1st week
Breast milk jaundice : 2nd week - 3rd month.

Racecadotril – Check enkephalinase inhibitor
↑ Na^+ and Cl^- absorption
↑ Stool consistency

Temperature

- Normal : 36.5 – 37°C
- Hypothermia : < 36°C
- Severe Hypothermia : < 32°C

	Neonatal Jaundice	EHBA – Extrahepatic Biliary Atresia
	Familial, intermittent	
USG	GB seen	GB not seen, Triangular cord sign (USG)
HIDA (Hepatobiliary Iminodiacetic Acid)	Decreased uptake Normal excretion	Normal uptake decreased excretion
Biopsy	Distortion of architecture	Bile duct proliferation periportal fibrosis

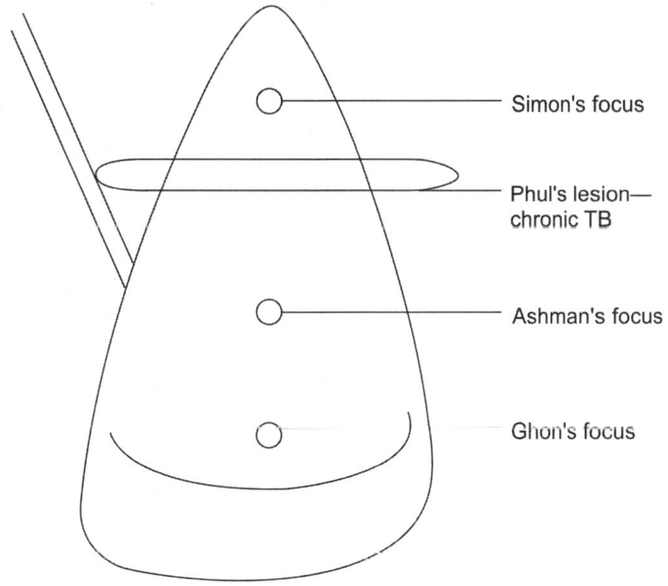

Congestive Cardiac Failure with Cardiomegaly

- MS – Mitral Stenosis
- TAPVC – Total Anomalous Pulmonary Venous Connection
- Cor triatriatum.

Craniosynostosis

- Dolichocephaly/scaphocephaly : Sagittal suture
- Brachycephaly : Coronal sutures
- Trigonocephaly : Metopic suture—pointed forehead
- Oxy/Acra/Terrencephaly : All sutures—turricephaly

Developmental Milestones

2 months	Social smile.
3 months	Neck holding, Recognizes mother, Cooing.
4 months	Grasp, Ring/rattle.
5 months	Sits with support, Bidextrous grasp/hold, Reaching objects, Mirror image, Mouthing, Babbling.
6 months	Roll over, Monosyllable, Sitting without support (6–8 min), Unidextrous/Palmar grasp, Transfer of object.
7 months	Stranger anxiety.
9 months	Standing with support, Pincer grasp, Bisyllable, Crawling.
10 months	Creeping, Bye-bye.
11 months	Cruising.
12 months	Walking with support towards parents.
13 months	Walking without support.
15 months	Spoon feeding with spills.
18 months	Running and climbing stairs, Speaks 10 words, Spoon feeding without spills.
15 months–18 months	Sphincter control.
2 years	Climbing steps by both feet, Draws line.
2.5–3 years	Name and sex.
3 years	Story, Dress on its own, Draws circle, Rides tricycle, Climbing steps by one foot, Knows name and sex.

Contd…

Contd...

4–5 years	Address and phone number.
4 years	Button on its own, Draws plus and square.
5 years	Draws triangle.
6 years	Draws diamond.

Human Milk

- Rich in Lactose (sweet)
- Rich in carbohydrates and proteins
- Increased Calcium and phosphate ratio
- Rich in essential fatty acid
- Fat and calorie are equal.

Human Milk

- Rich in vitamin K
- Rich in proteins
- Rich in solutes.

Breastfeeding Contraindicated in:

- MSUD (Maple syrup urine disease)
- Phenylketonuria (PKU)
- Lactose intolerance
- Galactosemia
- Anticancer
- Isoniazid (INH).

Chronic Myelogenous Leukemia (CML)—Juvenile

- Lymphadenopathy (enlarged)
- Spleen small
- Platelet decreased
- Monosomy 7
- Molecular mutations in BCR/ABL-**Negative,** i.e. **No mutation**.

Vesicoureteral Reflux

- **Surgery** (indication)
- Grade III/IV Bilateral— > 6 years
- Grade V Bilateral/scaring— > 1 year
- No surgery < 1 year.

Posterior Urethral Valve (PUV)—Males
Vesicoureteral reflux—80% female: Recurrent UTI

Bartter Syndrome—Type 4: SN Deafness:

- Hypokalemia
- Hypochlorine
- Hypercalciuria
- Increased renin
- Treatment: ACE inhibitor and NSAID.

Do Not Appear in Birth: LPS

L – Landau Reflex
P – Parachute (exists life long)
S – STNR–Symmetrical Tonic Neck Reflex

Day 1 Seizure – Metabolic: ↓Ca, glucose, pyridoxine.
Day 2/3 Seizure – CNS Trauma: SAH, SDH, IVH.
1st week Seizure – Aminoaciduria
Any time Seizure – Infection, Hyperthermia (HT), development defect of brain.

P-aminobenzoic acid (PABA) X Malaria

Lactoferrin X Escherichia coli (E. coli)

↑

Bifidus: in the intestinal flora of breastfed infants **Lactobacillus**

Lipase X Entamoeba

Peroxidase Glanders

VACCINE

- Typhoid Oral — > 6 years
- Vi capsular polysaccharide vaccine — > 2 years
- Whole cell.

Hep A > 2 years (0, 6)

Varicella > 1 year → <12 years schedule
Varicella > 1 year → >12 years 0, 1

Measles – TSST (toxic shock syndrome toxin-1)

BCG – NS

BCG, Measles, MMR – ILR top
OPV, Meases – Freezer

1st day OPV – Deep

BCG – Top

Varicella – 5 days before and 2 days after

DWARFISM

Constitutional

- Bone age < chronological age
- Bone age = Height age.

Functional

- Bone age = chronological age
- Bone age > Height age.

Hypopituitarism

Height age < Bone age < Chronological age.

ORS

WHO: Reduced osmolarity and Potassium equal.

ReSoMal (Rehydration Solution for Malnourished Children) Increased potassium equal.

Glycogen Storage Disease (GSD) – II : Heart-Pompe Disease

Glycogen Storage Disease (GSD) – IV : Cholesterolemia

Hypothyroidism

- True Macroglossia
- True precocious puberty
- Guthrie test—6th day heel prick TSH
- Disproportionate dwarfism.

Tuberous Sclerosis

- Hypopigmented 'ash leaf' patches
- Adenoma sebaceum (facial angiofibromas)
- Shagreen patches (subepidermal fibrosis).

Guillain-Barre Syndrome

Reflex – Lost first and gained last

First disease – Measles (Rubeola)

Second disease – Scarlet

Third disease – Rubella (Forchheimer spots)

Fourth disease – Filatow-Dukes' Disease (Atypical scarlet)

Fifth disease – Erythema infectiosum (slapped cheek syndrome)—Parvo virus

Sixth disease – Roseola infantum/Exanthem subitum—Nagayama's spots

Choreoathetosis

- **Wilson Disease** – **Wing beating tremor**
- **Hallervorden-Spatz Disease** – **Iron disease in Basal Ganglia**
- **Kernicterus – athetotic cerebral palsy (CP)** – **Status marmoratus**
- **Dyke-Davidoff-Masson syndrome (DDMS)** – In hemiplegic Cerebral palsy, atrophy of cortex and increase in ventricles size in hemisphere opposite to affected limb

Wilson Disease

- Avoid
- Shellfish
  - Chocolate
  - Nuts
  - Beef.

Atypical Febrile Seizure

- > 15 minutes (or) > 2 episodes of same febrile seizure
- Inappropriate arginine vasopressin (AVP) release
- Occurs between 3 months and 5 years.

Treatment

Clobazam (new).

Ataxia Telangiectasia

- Chromosome 11
- Oculomotor apraxia.

- **Lennox** – **Gastaut syndrome (LGS)—Lamotrigine**
- **Juvenile myoclonic** – **JANZ syndrome—*Treatment*: Valproate**
- **Infantile spasm** – **West syndrome—Vigabatrin/ACTH**
- **Tuberous sclerosis** – **Vigabatrin**
- **Miller Fisher syndrome** – **Guillain-Barré syndrome**:
  - External Ophthalmoplegia
  - Ataxia
  - Areflexia
  - anti-GQ1b IgG antibody.

Porencephaly : Cystic degeneration/Cavity lesions

Lissencephaly : Agyria

Schizencephaly

Holoprosencephaly

Trigonocephaly : Metopic suture, Pointed forehead

Oxycephaly/Turricephaly : Tower-shaped

Plagicephaly : Asymmetric fusion

Craniosynostosis

- Pfeiffer syndrome
- Apert syndrome
- Crouzon syndrome
- Carpenter syndrome
- Saethre-Chotzen syndrome (SCS).

HEAD CIRCUMFERENCE

- 35 cm + 2 cm/month for first 3 months
- 1 cm/month for next 3 months
- 0.5 cm/month for next 6 months.

Hot Cross Bun Appearance of Skull

Prominance of suture lines of skull and prominence of frontal and parietal eminences leading to 'bossing' of head in newborns. → **Rickets** and Congenital Syphilis.

Von Gierke's disease - Hepatosplenomegaly

- Doll facies
- Early morning fall/decrease in glucose causes seizures
- Pompe disease—Cardiomegaly.

Andersen Disease

Cardiomegaly, only with splenomegaly.

McArdle's Disease

- Burgundy-colored urine (myoglobinuria) after exercise (methemoglobinuria)
- Carnitine deficiency – Cardiomegaly.

- Fabry disease } AR/MR
- Mucopolysaccharidoses
- Gaucher's disease—Pericarditis

Phenylketonuria (PKU)

- 'Looks like angel, behaves like devil'
- Mousy odor urine
- Recurrent Vomiting
- Blood phenylalanine level increased after protein challenge (Breastfeeding).

Urine

- Sweet urine—isovaleric aciduria
- Tomcat urine odor—multiple carboxylase deficiency
- Rotten fish—trimethylaminuria.

Severe Chorea

Carbamazepine > Valproic acid > Haloperidol.

CCF

< 3 days	–	Atresia
1 week	–	TGA (Transposition of the great arteries), HLHS (Hypoplastic Left Heart Syndrome)
1–4 weeks	–	Coarctation of Aorta, TGA (Transposition of the great arteries)
1–2 months	–	TAPVC (Total anomalous pulmonary venous connection) ALCAPA (Anomalous left coronary artery from pulmonary artery) ECD (Endocardial cushion defect)

PDA

> 2 months—VSD, AS, PDA.

CHAPTER 18

Psychiatry

SYNDROMES IN PSYCHIATRY

Syndrome	Meaning
Cotart	Nihilistic delusion, world nothing
Ganser syndrome	Approximate answers, pseudodementia
De Clerambault	Erotomania
Capgras	Delusion of doubles
Fregoli	Various people are same
Folie a deaux	Induced or shared delusion
Ekbom syndrome	Restless leg syndrome
Gastaut Geshwind syndrome	High moral, hyposexuality, hypergraphic
Othello	Delusion of infidelity
Asperger syndrome	Professional speech, no mr
Retts syndrome	Only in girls, stereotyped hand moves, deceleration of head circumference
Kanner syndrome	Infantile autism
La belle indifference	Lack of concern towards symptom
Pisa syndrome	Tardive dystonia
Kleine-Levin	Increased sleep, increased appetite, increased sexual desire

Culture-bound Syndromes

Syndrome	Meaning
Koro	Penis shrinks
Dhat	Semen in urine
Latah	Automatic obedience
Piblokto	Eskimos in ice, tears dress
Whitligo	Believes that they are becoming monsters

Time Duration

Disorder	Time
Acute stress reaction	3 days
Adjustment disorder	< 3 months
PTSD	> 3 months

Contd…

Contd...

Depression	2 weeks
Dysthymia	> 2 years
Mania	1 week
Neuroleptic malignant syndrome	> 3 months
Pathological or morbid grief	> 6 months

NREM

Slow Wave/Orthodox Sleep

- Stage 4: Night terror, nocturnal enuresis, bruxism, sleep walking, sleep talking.

Frequency beta > alpha > delta

- Alpha: Awake, mind wandering, eyes closed
- Beta: Eyes open, awake
- Alpha disappearance: Onset of sleep
- Alpha reappearance: REM sleep.

REM

- Paradoxical sleep
- Reappearance of alpha
- Beta like activity
- Dreaming
- Atonia
- Rapid eye movement.

Narcolepsy

- Decreases REM latency
- Sleep attack, sleep paralysis, hypnagogic hallucinations
- Hypnogogic : Going to sleep
- Hypnopompic : On awakening

Other Causes of Reduced REM Latency

- Sleep deprivation and depression
- Cataplexy: Sleep paralysis
- Catalepsy: Waxy flexibility.

MEMORY TYPES

Implicit memory : Solve prolems, learn skills

Explicit memory : Declarative/facts storing

Jamais vu : Unfamiliarity of familiar

Déjà vu : Familiarity of unknown things.

TCA

Tricyclic

- Imipramine
- Amitriptyline
- Doxepin.

Tetracyclic

- Mianserin
- Amoxapine.

SNRI

- Venlaflaxin
- Duloxetine.

NDRI

- Bupropion.

NARI

- Reboxetine.

NSRI

- Thianeptin
- Amineptine.

SARI

- Trazadone
- Nefazodone.

NASSA

- Mirtazapine.

MAO I A

- Moclobemide
- Clorgyline.

MAO I B

- Selegiline.

No EPS

- Clozapine
- Trazadone
- Risperidone.

Fluoxetine : Longest Acting
Fluoxamine : Short Acting

Disorder	Time duration
Acute stress disorder	< 3 days
Adjustment disorder	< 3 months
PTSD	Within 6 months
Depression	2 weeks of symptoms
Mania	1 week of symptoms
Dysthymia	> 2 years of symptoms
Schizophrenia	1 month of clear-cut symptoms with 6 months of disturbances in social functioning, etc.

Freudian stage	Duration	Diseases associated
Oral	0–1	Schizo, mood disorder, alcoholism, dependent personality
Anal	1–3	OCD, coprophilia
Phallic	3–5	Hysteria, sexual deviation
Latency	6–11	Superego develops, neurotic disorders
Genital	11–13	Adult personality disorders

Type of memory	Characteristics
Episodic	Individual personal experiences, lost in amnesia
Semantic	Objects/people around
Implicit	Used for learning skills, solve problems (not a function if hippocampus)
Explicit	Facts storing

CHAPTER 19

Dermatology

DERMATOPHYTES

Trichophyton : Micro > macro—hair, skin, nails
Microsporum : Macro > micro, not nails
Epidermophyton : No micro, only macro—not in hair.

Alopecia

Noncicatricial

Localized

1. Alopecia arreata
2. Androgenic
3. Tinea capitis.

Generalized

1. Alopecia universalis
2. Ectodermal dysplasia.

Cicatricial

1. Lichen planus
2. Discoid lupus
3. Trauma
4. Basal cell carcinoma
5. Sarcoidosis
6. Linear scleroderma
7. Pseudopaladc.

Koebner's Phenomenon

1. Psoriasis
2. Lichen planus
3. DLE
4. Vitiligo
5. Wart
6. Molluscum
7. Kaposi sarcoma.

Pathergy

1. Bechet syndrome
2. Sweet syndrome
3. Pyoderma gangrenosum.

Purpura

- Palpable

Infective

1. Gonococcus
2. Meningococcus
3. Rocky mountain spotted fever.

Vasculitis (PHC)

1. PAN
2. HSP
3. Cryoglobulinemia.

Nonpalpable

1. ITP
2. DIC
3. Warfarin
4. Amyloid
5. Ehler danlos
6. Scurvy
7. Livedoid vasculitis
8. Monoclonal cryoglobulinemia
9. Wandelstorm hypergammaglobulinemia.

'THE CENTRALS'

Central crusting	Leishmaniasis
Central scaring	Lupus vulgaris
Central clearing	T. corporis

Bullous Disorder

Subcorneal

1. Bullous impetigo
2. Neutrophilic pustular dermatosis
3. Pemphigus foliaceuos
4. Miliaria crystalline
5. SSSS
6. IgA pemphigus.

Intraepidermal

1. Pemphigus vulgaris- intercellular IgG (fish net)
2. Paraneoplastic pemphigus
3. P. vegetans (variant of P. vulgaris) rare
4. P. erythematosis (variant of P. foliaceous)
5. Hailey hailey (familial benign pemphigus)
6. Darier disease (keratosis follicularis)
7. Incontinentia pigmenti
8. Miliaria rubra
9. Epidermolysis bullosa
10. Eczema
11. Insect bite, herpes.

Subepidermal

1. Bullous pemphigoid
2. Erythema multiforme
3. Dermatitis herpetiformis
4. Pemphigus gestations
5. Cicatricial pemphigus
6. Chr. bullous disorder of childhood
7. Linear IgA.

Granular

1. Erythema multiforme: IgG
2. Dermatitis herpetiformis: IgA microabscess
3. DLE (IgG C5 to 9).

- **Pemphigus** – Acanthocytes
- **Bullous pemphigoid** – Eosinophils
- **Dermatitis herpetiformis** – Eosinophils
- **Chr. bullous disorder of childhood** – PMN
- **Varicella/herpes** – Multinucleate giant cell

LEPRA REACTIONS

Borderline	Type 1 lepra reaction
Downgrading	Before treatment, lepromatous
Reversal	After treatment, tuberculoid

Ichthyosis

1. Ichthyosis vulgaris AD
2. Lamellar ichthyosis AR

3. Cong. Ichthyosiform erythroderma AR
4. X-linked ichthyosis (steroid sulphatase)
5. Ichthyosis nigra XR.

Leprosy

Indeterminate

1. Young school going
2. Endemic area
3. Always macule.

Tuberculoid

1. Active border
2. Asymmetrical
3. Feeding nerve.

Lepromatous

1. Symmetrical
2. Superciliary madarosis.

Borderline

BT

1. Satellite nodule
2. Asymmetrical.

BB

1. Inverted saucer.

BL

1. Symmetrical.

Indeterminate

1. Anesthetic
2. Endemic area.

Signs of Internal Malignancy

1. Bullous pemphigoid
2. Acquired ichthyosis
3. Erythema gyratumrepens (Ca bronchus)
4. Dermatomyositis
5. Annular erythema
6. Acanthosis nigricans (Ca stomach)
7. Erythema multiforme
8. Migratory neurolytic erythema
9. Palmoplantar keratoderma (Ca esophagus)
10. Pityriasis rotunda (Ca liver).

Wood's lamp—360 nm

Erythrasma	Coral red
Pseudomonas	Blue
Pityriasis versicolor	Apple green/golden yellow
Microsporum	Yellow
Porphyria cutanea tarda	Pinkish red
Tuberous sclerosis	Blue white
Freckles	Accentuated
Vitiligo	Total white

Syphilis

Bil. lymphadenopathy, painless, usually single ulcer with clear base with serous fluid, ***indurated***, bil. ***Nontender lypmphadenopathy.***

Donovanosis

Painless, multiple, margins elevated, ***beefy red ulcer***, bleed on touch, indurated, no, lymphadenopathy or ***pseudobubo*** (edema).

LGV

Painless, transient ulcer with tender ***unilateral painful lymphadenopathy*** (< one grp), ***groove sign***, esthiomene of vulva, stricture rectal.

Chancroid

Painful, multiple, ***bleeding ulcer*** with necrotic base with ***tender unilateral lymphadenopathy which may suppurate, undermined edge.***

Psoriasis

1. Auspitz sign
2. Grattage test
3. Burkley membrane
4. Munro Muller abscess
5. Wornoff ring.

Lichen Planus

1. Wickham striae
2. Civatte bodies
3. Sawtoothing
4. Pterygium nail
5. Max Joseph space
6. Basal degeneration
7. Lacy white
8. Mouth lesion.

NF

1. Lisch nodule > 2
2. Axillary freckling
3. Café au lait spots > 6
4. Neurofibromas > 2
5. Plexiform neurofibroma one or more.

Tuberous Sclerosis

1. Ash leaf macules earliest
2. Shagreen patch
3. Koenen tumor (periungual fibroma)
4. Adenoma sebaceum.

SWIMMING AND MEDICINE

Swimming pool granuloma	Mycobacterium marinum
Swimming pool conjunctivitis	Adenovirus/Chlamydia
Swimming pool veruccae	Plantar wart
Swimmer's itch	Schistosoma mansoni, schistoma japonicum

DLE

Central atropic, depigmented, surrounded by hyperpigmentation, coin-shaped, ***carpet track sign, treatment—chloroquine.***

Dermatitis Herpetiformis

Intensely pruritic, papules/vesicles/gluten sensitive, extensor involvement, ***IgA granular microabscess treatment—dapsone.***

Erythema Multiforme (Lyell Syndrome—TEN)

Herpes simplex, mycoplasma, symmetrical target lesion, palms and soles.

Incontinentia Pigmenti

X-linked dominant, Vesicle-wart-hyperpigmented-hypopigmented, starts in utero, dental and eye involvement, mutation in NFKB essential modulator. Called ***Bloch-Sulzberger syndrome.***

Lentigomaligna	***Least malignant***, elderly, face least common, Hutchinson's freckles
Nodular	***Most malignant***
Amelanotic	***Worst prognosis***
Superficial spreading	***Most common***
Acral lentiginous	Dark-skin Africans, ***sole***

Panniculitis

Type 4: Erythema nodosum (Miescher granuloma) infiltration of PMN—lymphocytes, eosinophils, septal panniculitis

Type 3: Erythema induratum—granulomatous, caseous necrosis, necrotizing vasculitis, lobar panniculitis, bazin (M. cheloni).

Weber-Christian: Relapsing nodular panniculitis.

Histiocytosis and Other Dermatological Conditions

Acute	Lotterer-Siwe
Chronic	Hand Schuller Christian
Kiguchi	Necrotizing histiocytic lymphadenitis
Sweet syndrome	Acute febrile neutrophilic dermatosis
Keratoacanthoma	Keratin plug, spontaneous regression, not premalignant
Actinic keratosis	Cutaneous horn, premalignant
Kimura	Eosinophilic dermatitis

CHAPTER

20 Orthopedics

TRACTION

Gallow, Bryant	Shaft femur #
Russel	Thochanteric #
Dunlop, Smith	Supracondylar # humerus
Perkins	Shaft of femur # adult
90-90	Shaft of femur # child
Head halter, crutchfield	Cervical spine #
Agnes hunt	Hip deformity correction
Well leg traction	Add, abd deformity of hip
Halo pelvic	Scoliosis
Bucks	Conventional skin traction

Splints

Bohler braun	Femur #
Aeroplane	Brachial plexus
Velpea/swathe	Shoulder dislocation
Von rosen, craig, pelvic harness	CDH
Mermaid splint	Rickets
Broomstick	Perthe
Velpea bandage, sling and swathe splint	Acromioclavicular dislocation

Pins

Steiman pin	Non osteoporotic bone
Denhams	Osteoporotic
Rush pin/nail	Intramedullary
Smith Peterson	Supracondylar femur

Braces

ASHE, Taylor	DS lumbar spine
SOMI	Cervical spine
Risser, noston, milwauker	Scoliosis

Cast

Hanging (sugar tong)	# humerus
Cylinder cast	# patella
PTB cast, Sarmiento	# tibia
Minerva	# cervical spine
Callot cast	Conjenital torticollis

Named Fractures

Robert jones	Avulsion # of base of 5th metatarsal
Monteggia	# proximal one third of ulna, dislocation of prox. radioulnar jt
Galeazzi	# distal third of radius dislocation of distal radioulnar jt
Esser lopressi	# radial head/neck with tearing of interroseus membrane
Barton	Distal articular # radius with distal radioulnar dislocation
Chauffeur	Radial styloid #
Bennet	Partial articular # first MC base with trapeziometacarpal dislocation
Rolando	Complete intraarticular # 1st MC base
Boxers	# neck of 5th MC
Night stick	# shaft of ulna
Corner	# lower third femur—battered baby syndrome
Straddle	Bil. pubic rami
Malgaigne	Pubic symphysis with SI joint
Bucket handle	Pubic symphisi with contralateral SI joint
Segond	Avulsion # lat. Tibial condyle
Potts	Bimaleolar
Cotton	Trimalleolar
Pilon	Lower articular surface tibia
Massonasi	Medial malleolus with # neck of fibula
Trilaux	Lower third of tibia
Avlators	Talus
Piplein	# head of femur
Gosselim	# of distal tibia
Jafferson	Burst # C1 atlas
Hangeman	Spondylolisthesis C2 over C3
Clay shoveller	Avulsion C7 spinous process
Chance	Through and through # vertebra
Tear drop	# dislocation vertebra, flexion compression force
Chopart	# dislocation intertarsal jt
Robert jones	Avulsion # base of 5th metatarsal
March	Stress # 2nd and 3rd metatarsal
Gaurdsman	Bil. mandibular condylar #
Motorcycle	Ring # base of skull

Contd...

Contd...

Blount disease	Infantile tibia vara
Caffy disease	Infantile cortical hypersteitis
Athletic pubalgia	Rectus abdominis
Students elbow	Olecranon bursitits
Housemaid knee	Prepatellar bursitis
Clergyman knee	Infrapatellar bursitis
Weavers	Ischial bursitis

Named Conditions

Mallet finger/baseball finger	Avulsion of ext. tenon of DP
Trigger finger	Flexor tenosynovitis at MCP joint
Skiers (game keepers) thumb	Ulnar collateral injury of MCP joint
Hammer toe	Plantar flexion of PIP joint
De quervian	Tenosynovitis of extensor pollicis brevis and abductor. pollicis longus
Rugger jersey finger	Avulsion of FDP
Coach finger	PIP dislocation
Caplan dislocation	MCP dislocation
Little leaguer elbow	Medial epicondyle avulsion
Sprangel shoulder	Failure of normal descent of scapula
Main en griffin	Claw hand- ulnar nerve
Pied en griffe	Claw toe- medial popliteal nerv e
Stove in hip	Acetabular #
Erb's palsy	Upper C5, C6
Klumpke's palsy	Lower T1 > C8
Tarsal tunnel syndrome	Post tibial nerve
Carpal tunnel syndrome	Median nerve
Cubital tunnel / guyon canal	Ulnar nerve
Thoracic outlet syndrome	C8T1
Meralgia paraesthesia	Lateral cutaneous nerve of thigh
Morton metatarsalgia	Interdigital nerve 3rd and 4th
Unhappy triad of O donoghue	MCL, ACL, medial meniscus

Classifications

Gustilo-Anderson	Compound #
Salter-Harris	Epiphyseal injury
Marvin Tile	# pelvis
Powel	# neck of femur
Garden	Medial trabecular stream
Lauge-Hansen	Ankle injury
Letournel	Acetabular #
Hawkins	Talus #
Sanders	Calcaneum
Mirel's criteria	Pathologic # > 7-prophylactic fixation

Osteochondritis

Kienbock	Lunate
Legg-Calve-Perthes	Femoral head
Kohler	Navicular
Panner	Capitulum
Islene	5th metatarsal base
Freiberg	2nd metatarsal head
Sheumann	Ring epiphysis of vertebral body
Osgood-Schlatter	Upper tibia
Sinding-Larsen-Johansson	Inferior pole patella
Sever (spur)	Calcaneum

Tumor

Epiphysis

1. Chondroblastoma
2. Osteoclastoma.

Diaphysis

1. Ewings sarcoma
2. Multiple myeloma
3. Eosinophilic granuloma
4. Enchondroma
5. Adamantinoma, fibrous dysplasia.

Bone Formation

1. ALP
2. Sr. osteocalcin
3. Sr. peptide type 1 procollagen.

Bone Resorption

1. Ur and Sr N and C telopeptide
2. Ur free dehydropuridinoline
3. Ur hydroxyproline
4. Ur hydroxulysine
5. TRAP TRAF
6. Sr. Sialoprotein.

CALCIFICATIONS

Disc calcification	Alkaptonuria
Chondrocalcinosis	Pseudogout
Periarticular calcification	Pseudogout
Ear pinna calcification	Addison's disease

Amputation

Midfoot

Lisfranc: Tarsometatarsal

Chopart: Mid tarsal.

Hindfoot

Syme: Distal tibia 0.6 cm from ankle joint

Sarmiento: Distal tibia 1.3 cm and malleoli

Boyd: Talectomy and calcaneotibial arthrodesis.

ORTHOTUMORS

1. **Multiple myeloma:** MC primary bone tumor, old age, vertebra, normal ALP, pathological #, raised ESR, anemia, renal failure with hypercalcemia.
2. **Osteosarcoma:** Can be secondry to Enchondromatosis, Fibrous dysplasia, osteoblastoma, Paget's disease and postirradiation. Lower end of femur—MC site. Sunray appearance and Codman triangle. Mayo regimen for treatment.
3. **Ewing's sarcoma:** <10 years, Diaphisis, t(11, 22), PAS positive, Diastase sensitive, melts like snow with radiotherapy but recurs, multicentric, presents with fever. Marcove Rosen regimen.
4. **Osteoclastoma** (Giant cell tumor)**:** Epiphysis, female, Enneking turn grafting, curettage can be done.
5. **Osteochondroma:** MC benign bone tumor, cartilaginous exostosis.
6. **Diaphyseal achalasias:** Autosomal dominant, short staure, trumpeting.
7. **Hemangioma:** Vertebra, polka dot sign in MRI, local gigantism.
8. **Osteoid osteoma:** Pain increased by alcohol, femur and double density sign.
9. **Chordoma:** Malignant, from notochord remnants, physaliferous cells.
10. **Chondrosarcoma:** Pelvis , huge mass, punctuate calcification.
11. **Osteoblastoma:** Pelvis, stippled calcification.
12. **Chondroblastoma:** Epiphysis, children, chicken wire calcification, Codman tumor.
13. **Fibrous dysplasia:** Mcune Albright syndrome, Ground glass opacity, Shepherd crook deformity.
14. **Fibrous cortical defect:** Non ossifying fibroma, developmental defect, metaphysis, tibia, cystic appearance, reduced intake in bone scan.
15. **Unicameral bone cyst:** Humerus, Trap door or Fallen fragment sign.
16. **Aneurysmal bone cyst:** Proximal tibia, transverse process, cortex breached, Blister bone sign, Pencil in cup.
17. **Adamantinoma:** Mandible > tibia, ameloblastoma.
18. **Enchondroma:** Ollier's disease, Maffucci syndrome metacarpal and metatarsal bones.
19. **Synovioma:** t (X, 18) spotty calcification, lymphatic spread.

Achondroplasia

- FGFR—3 mutation
- In increased paternal age
- Disproportionate dwarfism
- Trident hand—short equal sized fingers, gap between middle and ring finger

- Champagne glass pelvis
- Lumbar canal stenosis.

Osteopetrosis

- Marble bone disease
- Alber Schonberg disease
- Decreased osteoclastic activity
- Increased bone density
- Carbonic anhydrase II deficiency
- Rugger Jersy spine
- Osteomyelitis of jaw
- Candle wax dribbling
- Erlermayer flask deformity.

Paget's Disease

- Ostetis deformans
- Old age
- Slow virus—Paramyxovirus suspected
- Only ALP is increased, Sr Calcium normal
- Cotton wool spot in skull
- Ivory vertebra
- Platybasia and leonine facies
- Deafness
- Hyperdynamic circulation and heart failure.

CHAPTER

21

Radiology

VIEWS

Caldwell	Occipitofrontal—SOF, foramen rotendum, lamina papyracea
Waters	Sinuses, orbital floor
Towne	Petrosal region, pyramid, pineal gland
Stenver	Ear
Transorbital	Int. auditory canal
Rhees	Optic canal
Basal	Sphenoid, zygoma, mandibular condyle
Oblique	Orbital rim
Laws	Mastoid
Odontold	C1C2
RAO	Lt. atrium, GB, mitral valve
LAO	Tracheal bifurcation
Lordotic	Apex, lingula, lat. sulcus
Reverse lordotic	Interlobar effusion
Lat.decubitus	Min. pleural effusion
Strikers	Recurrent dislocation of shoulder
Skyline	# patella
Rib hump	Scoliosis
Frog leg	Perthes
Barlow proj	CDH
Orthopantomogram	Tooth, mandible, condyles, styloid process
Sunset view	Femoropatellar dysplasia

Investigations of Choice

Aortic dissection	MRI
Aortic aneurysm	CT angiogram
Pulm. embolism	CT angio D dimer
Renal artery stenosis	MRA
Pheochromocytoma	MRI > MIBG
Space occupying lesion	MRI with gadollinum

Contd…

Contd...

Avascular necrosis	MRI
Stress #	MRI Bone scan—earliest sensitive
Diffuse axonal injury	MRI
Cavernous hemangioma liver	MRI
Head injury/acute bleed	Plain CT
JNA	Contrast CT
ILD Bronchiectasis Pancreatitis Diverticulitis	CT
Diverticulosis	Barium enema
Interval angina	Arteriography
SMA syndrome	Contrast CT
GIST initial Recurrent/response to treatment	CECT PET
PNET	Somatostatin scintigraphy
Insulinoma	Endoscopic USG
Parathyroid adenoma	Fuscin scan (MIBG + CT)
Focal nodular hyperplasia	Colloid scintigraphy
Air embolism	TO echo
Meniscal injury	Arthroscopy > MRI
Bile duct Injury/leak Stricture	 CT-ERCP/PTC CT-MRCP/PTC

- Ionizing and damaging power: $\alpha > \beta >$ X-rays $> \gamma$
- Penetration power: $\gamma >$ X-rays $> \beta > \alpha$

- Minimum fluid: USG
- Minimum air: CT.

Radiodense

- Chloral hydrate
- Heavy metals
- Iron
- Phenothiazine
- Salicylates.

DTPA

- Renal function
- Renal transplant
- Obstruction
- Renal HT.

Teletherapy: Cs137 and Co60

Ground Glass Appearance

- HMD
- TAPVC
- Alveolar proteinosis
- Allergic alveolitis
- Interstitial lymphoma.

Eggshell Calcification

- TB
- Histoplasmosis
- Coccidomycosis
- Silicosis
- Sarcoidosos
- Lymphoma.

Air Bronchogram

- Pneumonia
- Alveolar cell CA
- Kaposi sarcoma
- Lymphoma
- Pulm. infarction
- Pulm. edema
- Fat embolism
- Metastasis.

Miliary Mottling

- TB
- Brucella
- Fungal infections
- Varicella
- Loeffler
- Ca alveolar, lymphoma, lung
- Pulmonary edema
- Pulmonary Fibrosis
- Pneumoconiosis
- Sarcoidosis
- RA
- HMD.

X-RAY APPEARANCES IN CHD

ASD	Great hilar dance
Primary pulm. HT	Jug handle
Reverse	Coarctation of aorta

Contd...

Contd…

TOF	Coeur en sabot
D_TGA	Egg on side
L_TGA	Smooth left heart border
Uncorrected TGA	Apple on string
Persistent truncus arteriosus	Sitting duck
Tricuspid atresia	Great box

CHAPTER 22

Anesthesiology

Depolarizing	Nondepolarizing
S. choline	dTC (bp falls)
Decamethonium	Curoniums (pancuronium maintains bp)
	Curiums (releases histamine)
	Gallamine

Phase 1 block is increased by – Isoflurane, Mg, Li, Anti-ChE

Phase 2 block is increased by – Enflurane and reversed by Anti-ChE.

Fastest acting muscular blockers	S.Ch, Rapacurium and Rocuronium
Shortest acting muscle blockers	S.Ch, Mivacurium
Longest acting blockers	Pipecuronium and doxacurium

Succinyl Choline

- C/I in myopathy due to increased K +
- Muscle soreness +
- Dual block (phase 1 and 2)
- Increases IOP
- Malignant HTN +

Gallamine

- C/I in RF
- Teratongenic
- Most sensitive to myasthenia.

Vecuronium

Least histamine relase but can exacerbate asthma.

Droperidol

- D2 blockade
- Reduces BP
- Catatonia +

Ketamine

- NMDA antagnonist
- Dissociative anesthesia and complete analgesia
- Bronchodilator
- DOC in Obst Hghe, Shock, Full stomach, children
- Hallucination can be treated with lorazepam.

Thiopentone

- Hyperalgesia
- Reduces ICT and seizure threshold
- Causes RR depression and bronchoconstriction
- C/I in porphyria
- DOC in thyrotoxicosis.

Propofol

- Reduces airway reflex: Useful in bronchoscopy
- Day care surgery: Very useful
- Antiemetic
- Reduces ICT and seizure threshold
- Safe in porphyria and HTN
- Reduce CO, PVR and BP
- **PRIS:** Metabolic acidosis, MODS, rhabdomyolysis, hepatomegaly.

Etomidate

- GABA-A agonist
- Cardiostable
- C/I in porphyria
- Causes vitamin c deficiency
- Adrenal suppression + due to 11 beta OHlase block.

Neuroleptic Anesthesia

- Fentanyl
- Droperidol
- N_2O.

TIVA

- Propofol
- Remafentanyl.

Malignant HTN

Causes/contraindicated	DOC
S.Ch	Propfol
Ether	Procaine
Cyclopropane	N2O
Halothane	Ketamine
Flurane	Thipentone
Amide LA	Barbituates
TCA	Pancuronium
MAO inhibitors	
Phenothiazines	

Intracranial Tension

Increased	Ketamine, halothane
Decreased	Thiopentone, Propofol, Droperidol, Etomidate

Myasthenia

- S. Ch
- Propofol
- Isoflurane
- Cisatracurium/Atracurium
- Mivacurium
- Rapacurium.

Balanced Anesthesia

- Thiopentone: Induction
- Curare: Relax
- N2O: Amnesia
- Meperidine: Analgesia.

Anesthetics and Asthma

Vecuronium, Ketamine, Halothane, Ether.

Gas	Cylinder (Body, shoulder)	PIN index
O_2	Black, white	2, 5
CO_2	Grey, grey	1, 6
N_2O	Blue, blue	3, 5
Entanox	Black + white, blue	7
Halothane	Amber	
Cyclopropane	Orange	3, 6
Thiopentone	Yellow	

NO SODALIME (CT SCA'M').

Chloroform, Trielene, Sevoflurane (Compound A), Methoxyflurane

RUBBER TUBE EROSION: Halothane (metal also), Methoxyflurane.

Maximum and Minimum

	Maximum		Minimum
MAC	N2O	**MAC**	Methoxyflurane (most potent)
BGC	Methoxyflurane (slowest)	**BGC**	Desflurane (fastest)

DAY CARE ANESTHETICS

(Dr. Manmohan Singh is a Prime Minister)

Desflurane, midazolam, S. Ch, Isoflurane, Alfentanyl, Propofol, Mivacurium.

Mapleson Classification

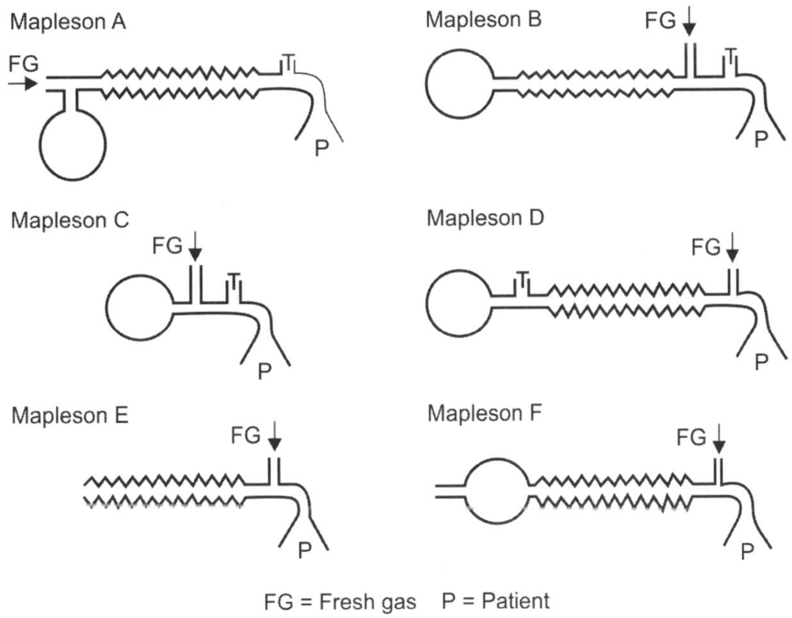

Fig. 22.1: Mapleson Classification

A - Magill and lack

B - High flow

C - High flow, B and C are not so useful for anesthesia, more for resuscitation

D - Bain modified

E - Ayre's T piece

F - Jackson-Rees medication of E, E and F are valveless.

Appendix 1

MISNOMERS

- Histoplasma capsulatum : Not capsulated
- White bile : Not white, not bile, its mucous
- Malignant otitis media : Not malignant
- Mycosis fungoides : Not a fungal infection/ t cell lymphoma
- Mycotic aneurysm : Not fungal but bacterial
- Amanita muscarii : Not muscarinic
- Lupus anticoagulant : Causes thrombosis
- Botyryomycosis : Caused by staph
- Compound palmar ganglion : Not a ganglion, its due to TB
- Herpangina : Not angina, caused by coxsackie.

TRIADS

Triad of Alport's Syndrome

- Sensorineural deafness
- Progressive renal failure
- Ocular anomalies

Triad of Behçet's Syndrome

- Recurrent oral ulcers
- Genital ulcers
- Iridocyclitis
- *[Mnemonic: Cannot see, cannot pee, cannot eat spicy curry]*

Beck's Triad

- Muffled heart sound
- Distended neck veins
- Hypotension.

Charcot's Triad

- Pain
- Fever
- Jaundice.

Gradenigo's Triad

- Sixth cranial nerve palsy
- Persistent ear discharge
- Deep seated retro orbital pain.

Triad of Hypernephroma

- Pain
- Hematuria
- Renal mass.

Hutchinson's Triad

- Hutchinson's teeth
- Interstitial keratitis
- Nerve deafness.

Triad of Kwashiorkor

- Growth retardation
- Mental changes
- Edema

Saint's Triad

- Gallstones
- Diverticulosis
- Hiatus hernia.

Trotter's Triad

- Conductive deafness
- Immobility of homolateral soft palate
- Trigeminal neuralgia.

Virchow's Triad

- Stasis
- Hypercoagulability
- Vessel injury.

Whipple's Triad

- Hypoglycemia during attacks
- S. glucose 10%
- Hypergammaglobulinemia
- Lytic bone lesions.

Hemolytic Uremic Syndrome Triad

- Anemia
- Thrombocytopenia
- Renal failure.

Fanconi Syndrome Triad

- Aminoaciduria
- Proteinuria
- Phosphaturia.

Tetany in Children–Triad

- Stridor
- Carpopedal spasm
- Convulsions.

Alkaptonuria Triad

- Ochronotic arthritis
- Ochronotic pigmentation
- Urine darkens on standing.

Anderson Triad

- Bronchiectasis
- Cystic fibrosis
- Vitamin A deficiency.

Triad of Albinism *[BADS]*

- Black locks
- Occulocutaneous Albinism
- Deafness of sensorineural type.

Pentad of TTP

- Microangiopathic hemolytic anemia
- Fever
- Disturbed neurological function
- Renal failure
- Thrombocytopenia.

Triad of Causes of Biotin Deficiency

- Glossitis
- Alopecia
- Dermatitis.

Reynolds' Pentad

- Abdominal pain
- Fever
- Jaundice
- Shock, and altered sensorium

Pentalogy of Fallot

- Fallot's tetralogy with, in addition, a patent foramen ovale
- Atrial septal defect.

Triple Test

- Estimation of hcg
- Estriol, and AFP.

O'Donoghue Triad

- Medial collateral ligament
- Anterior cruciate ligament
- Medial meniscus.

MacDonald's Triad (ASPD)

- Enuresis
- Firesetting
- Animal cruelty.

Cushing Triad of Raised ICP

- Bradycardia
- Bradypnea
- Hypertension.

Hemobilia—Triad of Sandblom

- Malena
- Obstructive jaundice
- Biliary colic [MOB]

Kartagener's Syndrome Triad

- Triad of bronchiectasis
- Recurrent sinusitis
- Situs inversus.

Pentalogy of Cantrell (XLD)

- Lower thoracic wall malformations [cleft sternum]
- Ectopia cordis
- Epigastric omphalocele
- Anterior midline diaphragmatic hernia
- Cardiac anomalies.

Beck's Triad

- Kussmaul's sign
- Pulsus paradoxus
- Muffled heart sound.

Atta's Traid in Bilharzial Dysentery

- Bleeding per rectum
- Polyposis
- Clubbing of fingers.

Saint's Triad

- Gall stones
- Diverticulosis
- Hiatal hernia.

Meltzer's Triad (Cryoglobinemia)

- Palpable purpura
- Myalgia
- Arthralgia.

NEWER DRUGS

Drugs	Notes
Rifamycin	UTI in Pregnancy
Spectinomycin	Gonorrhea in Pregnancy
Aztreonam (a monobactam)	When aminoglycosides are contraindicated Safe in pregnancy Can be used in UTI, allergy, against gram negative bacilli
Daptomycin	Persistance Diptheria, Vancomycin Resistant Enterococcus (VRE) Vancomycin Resistant Staphylococcus aureus (VRSA) Methicillin Resistant Staphylococcus aureus (MRSA) Antagonises surfactant – *cannot be* used in Pneumonia
Retapamulin	Inhibits 50S Methicillin susceptible Impetigo (Staph and Strep)
Tetrabenazine	Dopamine depletor Used in Huntington's Disease
Rotigotine	Non ergot Dopamine agonist
Alvimopan [M-Morphine A-Anagonist]	Peripherally acting *μ-opioid antagonist* used in *postoperative ileus*
Istaroxime	Positive inotropic agent, inhibition of sodium/potassium adenosine triphosphatase Na+/ K+ ATPase (Like digoxin) Lusitrophy – increased myocardial relaxation
Omapatrilat	Vasopepidase inhibitor Increases BNP Brain Natriuretic Polypeptide
Enoximone	Phosphodiesterase IIIa inhibitor
Levosimendan	Increases Myocardial Calcium Sensitivity Phosphodiesterase inhibitor
Ecadotril	*Neutral endopeptidase* inhibitor (NEP) CCF
Indacrinone	Decreases reabsorption of *uric acid* is a *loop diuretic.* Used in patients of *gout* with *hypertension*
Aliskiren	Direct *renin inhibitors*
Anakinra	Is an interleukin-1 (IL-1) receptor antagonist used in Septic shock and Rheumatoid arthritis
Diacerein	*Interleukin-1 beta* receptor antagonist DMARD
Oprelvekin	Recombinant interleukin eleven (IL-11) increased platelet production.

Contd…

Contd…

Aldesleukin	Interleukin 2 (IL-2) Used in RCC and Malignant melanoma
Molsidomine	*Newer Nitrate* and no tolerance against it long acting *vasodilating drug.*
Vernakalant	Recent atrial fibrillation → Sinus rhythm Multiple ion channel blocker
Ezetimibe	Lowers plasma *cholesterol* levels Blocks NPC1L1 (Niemann-Pick C1-like 1) protein
Avasimibe	Inhibitor of acyl coenzyme A-cholesterol acyltransferase 1 (ACAT-1)
Torcetrapib	*Cholesterylester transfer protein* (CETP) inhibitor increases HDL levels
Exemestane	Irreversible aromatase inhibitors
Romidepsin	*Histone deacetylase* inhibitor as a treatment for cutaneous T-cell lymphoma (CTCL)
Vorinostat	*Histone deacetylase* inhibitor as a treatment for cutaneous T-cell lymphoma (CTCL)
Bexarotene	A *retinoid* as a treatment for cutaneous T-cell lymphoma (CTCL)
Defibrotide	To treat Veno-occlusive disease of liver especially caused by alkylating agents
Amifostine	Detoxifies reactive metabolites of platinum and alkylating agents, used to decrease the cumulative nephrotoxicity reduces severe oral mucositis
Palifermin	Recombinant keratinocyte growth factor(KGF) reduces severe oral mucositis
α-**Tocopherol**	Is a cardioprotective agent Is a free radical scavenger Reduces cardiotoxic side effects of anthracyclines
Dexrazoxane	Is a cardioprotective agent Is an iron chelator Is a free radical scavenger Reduces cardiotoxic side effects of anthracyclines
Fulvestrant [Fulv *est r ant*]	Is a Pure estrogen receptor antagonist Is a selective estrogen receptor down-regulator (SERD)
Aprepitant	Neurokinin 1 (NK_1) receptor antagonist used in Cisplatin (chemotherapy) induced vomiting is a substance P antagonist.
Rasburicase	*Urate oxidase* (an *enzyme* that metabolizes *uric acid* to *allantoin*) Used in chronic gout
Mesna	Sodium 2-sulfanylethanesulfonate (name of the substance is an acronym for 2-**me**rcapto**e**thane **s**ulfonate **Na**)
Romiplostim	Platelet stimulating peptide Used inchronic idiopathic (immune) thrombocytopenic purpura(ITP)
Eltrombopag	Oral thrombopoietin Used in thrombocytopenia Aplastic anemia (FDA February 2014)
Filgrastim	A granulocyte colony-stimulating factor (G-CSF) analog
Sargramostim	Is a *recombinant granulocyte macrophage colony-stimulating factor* (GM-CSF)
Danaparoid	A heparinoid used in DVT and *heparin-induced thrombocytopenia* (HIT)
Abciximab	A glycoprotein IIb / IIIa receptor antagonist
Tirofiban	A glycoprotein IIb / IIIa receptor antagonist
Eptifibatide	A glycoprotein IIb / IIIa receptor antagonist
Daltroban	Thromboxane A2 receptor antagonist
Dazoxiben	Thromboxane synthase inhibitor

Contd…

Contd…

Cilostazol	A *phosphodiesterase inhibitor* inhibits platelet aggregation to relieve claudication pain in PVD
Dipyridamole	A *phosphodiesterase inhibitor* increasing cellular cAMP levels inhibits platelet aggregation
Thioctic acid / α-lipoic acid	Treatment for Amanita phalloides (APL) *mushroom poisoning*
Prenalterol	β_1- adrenergic agonist a *cardiac stimulant*
Dronabinol	A cannabinoid *anti emetic* properties
Loxiglumide	*Cholecystokinin (CCK) antagonist* used in constipation
Plicamycin	Used in Paget's disease of bone Decreases blood Calcium (rarely, in management of *hypercalcemia*)
Racecadotril	Enkephalinase inhibitor an *antidiarrheal* drug
Apafant [A *paf* *ant*]	*P*latelet *A*ctivating *F*actor (PAF) receptor *ant*agonist Its first clinical target is acute pancreatitis.
Licofelone	A dual *COX / LOX* inhibitor A disease-modifying OA drug (DMOAD)
Teriparatide	Recombinant form of parathyroid hormone (PTH) treatment of *osteoporosis*
Cinacalcet	A *calcimimetic* decreases parathyroid hormone (PTH) treatment of *secondary hyperparathyroidism*
Xantinol nicotinate	A vasodilator used in Buerger disease
Oxerutin	Lymphedema
Saxitoxin	A selective *sodium channel blocker.* Is a neurotoxin à paralytic shellfish toxin (PST)
Dexmedetomidine	Is an *agonist* of *α_2-adrenergic receptors* used as preanesthetic agent
Indoramin	Is an *alpha-1*selective adrenoceptor antagonist used in Hypertensive emergensies
Apazone	Has uricosuric properties a NSAID
Ceftobiprole	Is a fifth-generation *cephalosporin antibiotic*
Bithionol	An *antihelmintic* used to treat *Fasciola hepatica* (liver flukes)
Prasugrel	Is a P2Y12 inhibitor (of ADP Block) used as oral antiplatelet agent and in coronary stent
Tapentadol	Centrally acting *opioid analgesic* dual mode of action as μ-opioid receptor anagonist and as a nor epinephrine (NE) reuptake inhibitor
Mecasermin	Is *recombinant* human *insulin-like growth factor 1* (IGF-I)
Probucol	Inhibits the oxidation of cholesterol in LDLs
Lacosamide	Blocks collapsin response mediator protein 2 (CRMP-2) used in partial seizures

Appendix 2

PHYSIOLOGY

Renal plasma flow

$$RPF = \frac{\mu V}{P}$$

Renal blood flow

$$RBF = RPV \times \frac{1}{1-HCT} \text{ and } RPV = \text{Renal plasma volume}$$

$$\text{Free water clearance} = V - \frac{\mu v}{p}$$

Effective renal plasma flow

$$ERPF = \frac{\mu v}{P_{(PAH)}} - 625 \text{ mL/min}$$

$$\text{Actual renal plasma flow} = \frac{ERPF}{ER} - 700 \text{ mL/min}$$

$$ER = \frac{SR_{AC} - SR_{VC}}{SR_{AC}}$$

μ – Concentration of creatinine in urine
v – Volume of urine
p – Concentration of creatinine in plasma

$$\text{Velocity} = \frac{V_{max} \times [s]}{K_m + [s]}$$

$$LDL = \text{Total cholesterol} - HDL + \frac{TGL}{5}$$

$$\text{Serum osmolality} = \frac{\text{Glucose}}{18} \times 2\,(Na^+) + \frac{BUN}{2.8}$$

$$\text{Total body water} = \text{Plasma volume} \times \frac{100}{100 - PCV}$$

$$PAO_2 = FiO_2 \times (P_\beta - P_{H_2O}) - \frac{PaCO_2}{R}$$

P_β – Atmospheric pressure – 760
P_{H_2O} – Partial pressure of water – 47
R – Respiratory quotient

Respiratory Quotient

$$R = \frac{CO_2 \text{ output}}{O_2 \text{ uptake}}$$

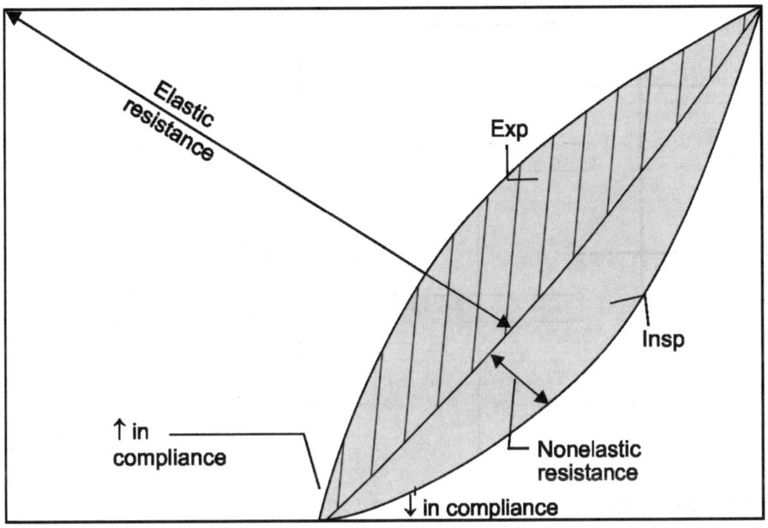

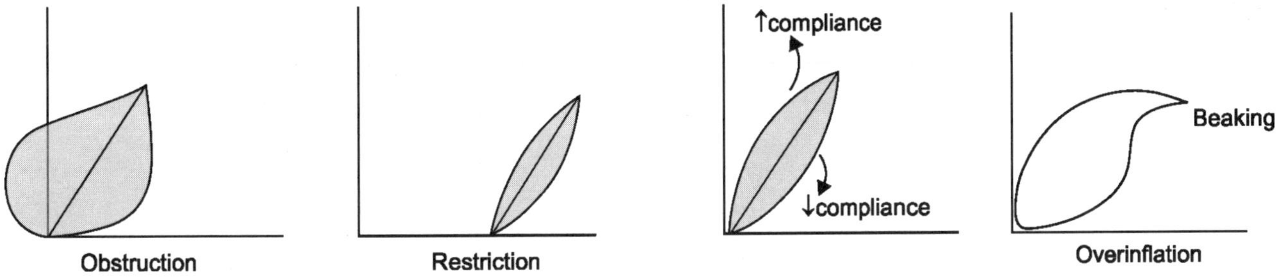

Lung:

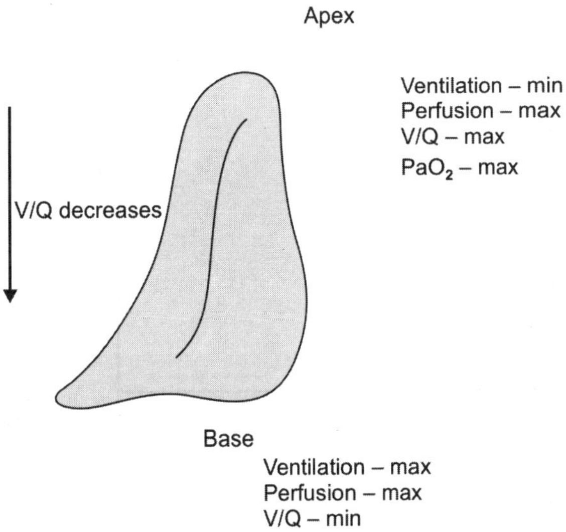

Sarcomere: Arrangement:

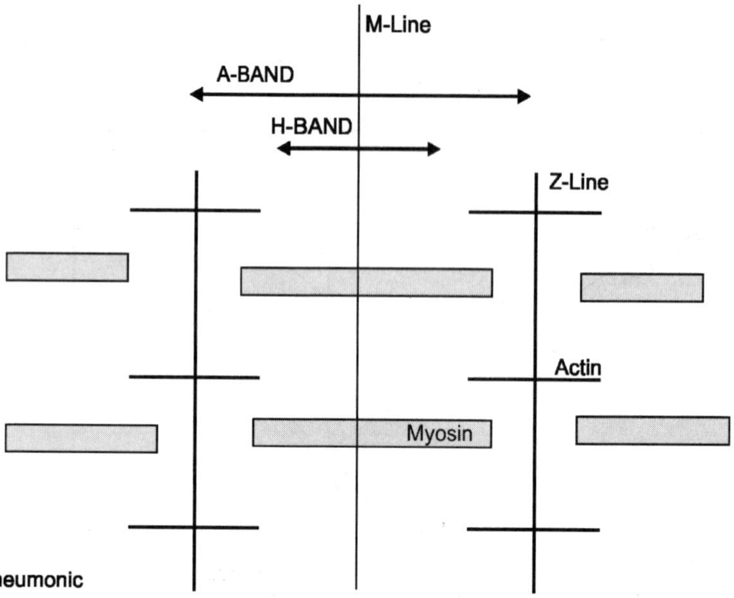

Pneumonic

AHM (Assistant Headmaster)

During contraction

H — Disappears
A — Constant

Cerebellum:

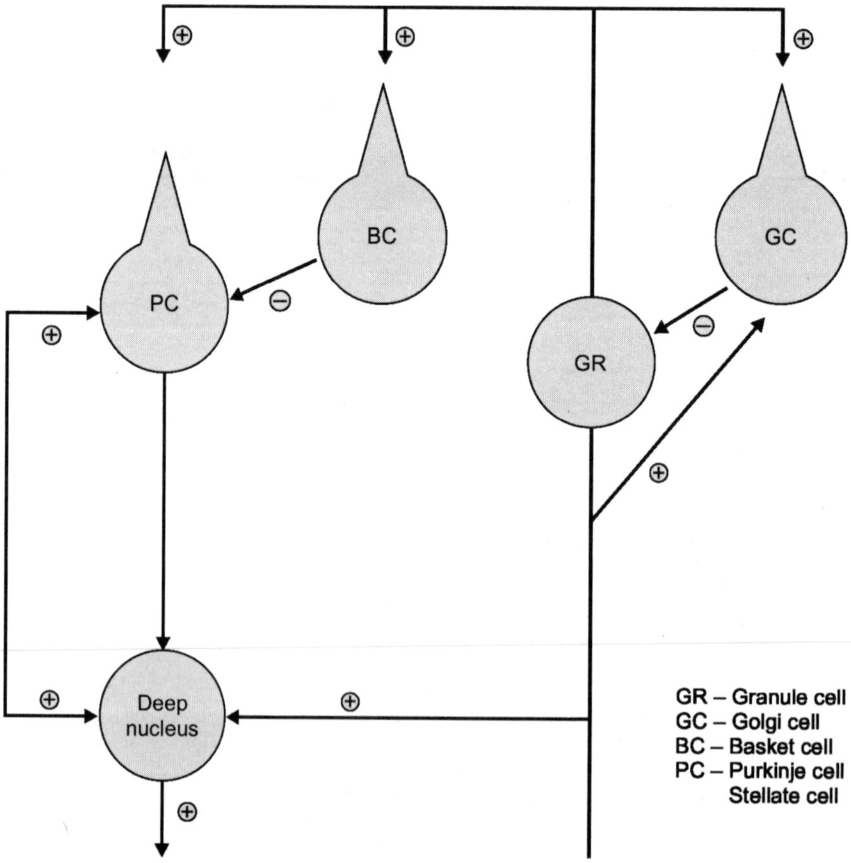

Bag and Plate:

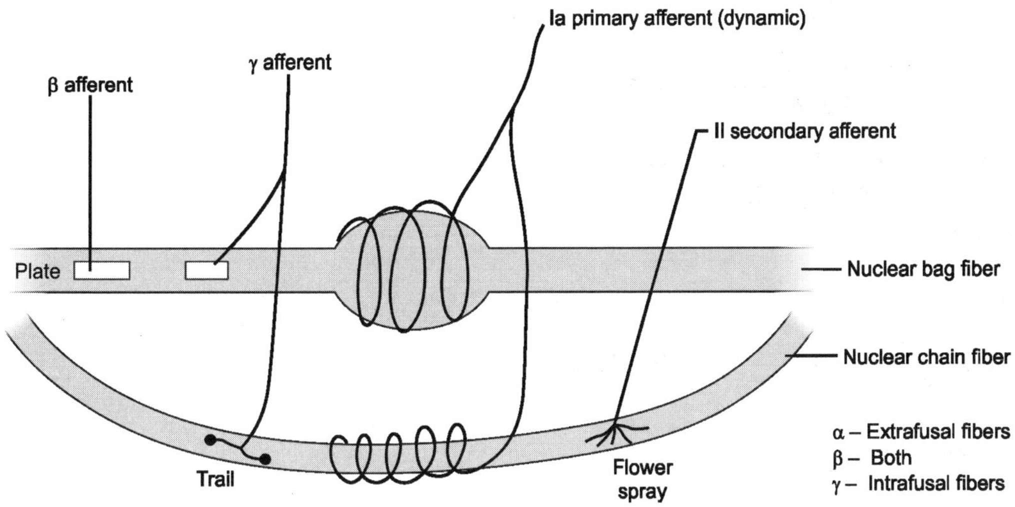

Laplace Low

Sphere $P = \frac{2T}{\gamma}$ T – Tension, γ – Radius

Cylinder $P = \frac{T}{\gamma}$

Reynold Number

$Re = \frac{PDV}{\eta}$ P – Density
D – Diameter
η – Viscocity

Hagen-Poiseuille law

$R = \frac{8L\eta}{\pi\gamma^4}$ κ – Resistance to flow
L – Length
η – Viscocity

$NFP = k\,[(P_C - p_\iota) - (\pi_C - \pi_i)]$
π – Colloid concotic pressure
P – Hydrostatic pressure
ι – Interstitial pressure
C – Capillary pressure

Creatine Clearance

$GFR = \frac{140 - Age \times w + (kg)}{72 \times cr}$ – Male

Female × 0.8

$\text{Venous Return} = \frac{MSFP - RAP}{RVR}$

Fick Principle

$\text{Cardiac output: } CO = \frac{O_2 \text{ Consumption}}{A\text{–}VO_2 \text{ difference}}$

Cardiac index: $CI = \frac{\text{Cardiac output}}{\text{BSA}} = 3.2\ L/m^2/min$

$$\text{Ejection fraction} = \frac{(LVEDD)^3 - (LVESD)^3}{(LVEDD)^3} \times 100$$

LVEDD – Left ventricle end diastolic diameter
Alveolar Ventilation = TV – DV × RR
TV – Tidal volume
DV – Dead space
RR – Resp rate

$\text{Dysinoeic Index} = \frac{BR}{MVV} \times 100$ Be – Breath rate

< 60 – Dyspnea

MVV – RMV = BR

Pharmacology

5 $t^1/_2$ = Steady state concentration
Loading dose = V_d × Target concentration
Vd – Volume of distribution

$$\text{Maintenance dose} = \frac{\text{Dosing rate} \times \text{Dosing interval}}{\text{F (Bioavailability)}}$$

Or

Clearance × Target concentration

$$\text{Volume of Distribution (Vd)} = \frac{\text{Dose administered}}{\text{Plasma conc.}}$$

Bioavailability F = f (1 – ER) ER = Extraction ratio

$t^1/_2 = 0.7 \times \frac{V}{CL}$ CL – clearance

Biochemistry Formula

Fatty acid oxidation:

$$\text{No. of ATT} = \left[\frac{(n-2)}{2} \times (5)\right] + \left[\frac{n}{2} + 12\right] - 2$$

(5) – β oxidation
(2) – TCA cycle
2 ATP less per double bond fatty acid

$$\left[\frac{(n-2)}{2} \times 4\right] + \left[\frac{n}{2} \times 10\right] - 2$$

If specific, then $NADH_2 = 2.5$
$FADH_2 = 1.5$

$FADH_2$ = 2 ATP (2.5 accurate specific)
$NADH_2$ = 3 ATP (1.5 specific)

Number of ATPs

- Cytric acid cycle (TCA) = 12 (10) specific
- Glycolysis – Aerobic = 8 (7)
  – Anaerobic = 2
- Pyruvate dehydrogenase complex = b
- Glucose by aerobic glycolysis
- Glucose burning in muscle = 36 (Gly – 3 PO_4 SHUTTLE)
- Gluconeogenesis uses 6 ATP
- Purine synthesis – 4 ATP + 2 AMP
- Urea – 3 ATP

Reticulocyte Correction Index

$$RI = \frac{\text{Reti count}}{2} \times \frac{\text{Hb}}{\text{Normal Hb}}$$

Absolute Reticulocyte Count

$$ARC = \frac{RI}{100} \times RBC$$

$$\text{Transferrin saturation} = \frac{\text{Sr. Iron}}{\text{TIBC}} \times 100$$

$$\text{Mentzer Index} = \frac{MCV}{RBC}$$

> 13 – Iron deficiency
> 13 – Thalassemia
Red Cell Distribution > 13 – Iron deficiency
Width
RDW

$$\text{RDW Index} = \frac{MCV \times RDW}{RBC}$$ > 220 – Iron deficiency
< 220 – Thalassemia

$$\text{Volume of well} = \frac{3.14 \times d^2 \times h}{4} \times 1000$$

2g of Bleeching powder for 455 liters of water

$$TDI = \frac{\text{NOEL/LOAEL}}{\text{UF}}$$

$$\text{Guideline value GV} = \frac{\text{TDI} \times \text{body wt} \times \text{P(\% of TDI)}}{C}$$ P – Percentage of TDI

C – Consumption

$$\text{Quetelet Index (BMI)} = \frac{\text{Wt (kg)}}{\text{Ht}^2\text{ (m)}}$$

$$\text{Ponderal Index} = \frac{\text{Ht (cm)}}{Y_3 \sqrt{\text{wt}}} \text{ or } \frac{\text{Wt (g)}}{(\text{Ht})^3}$$

< 2 – asymmetric IUGR
> 2 – symmetric IUGR

$$\text{Pear Index} = \frac{\text{Total no. of accidental pregnancy} \times 1200}{\text{No. of patients} \times \text{No. of months observed}}$$

$$\text{Protein-Efficiency Ratio} = \frac{\text{Weight increase (g)}}{\text{Protein consumption (g)}}$$

$$\text{Not Protein Utilization (NPU)} = \frac{\text{Retained } N_2}{N_2 \text{ in food}} \text{ or } \frac{\text{Digestibility coefficient} \times \text{Biological value}}{100}$$

$$\text{Biological value} = \frac{\text{Retained } N_2}{\text{Absorbed } N_2}$$

Brocas Index = Ht (cm) – 100

$$\text{Lorentz Formula} = \text{Ht (cm)} - 100 - \frac{\text{Ht (cm)} - 150}{.2\text{ (F) or } 4\text{(M)}}$$

$$\text{Corpulence Index} = \frac{\text{Actual weight}}{\text{Desirable weight}} \text{ – should be} < 2$$

Hardy-Weinberg Law of population genetics
$p^2 + 2pq + q^2 = 1$
Nondysfunction = (2n + 1), (2n – 1)
Anaphase log = (2n), (2n – 1)

Statistics

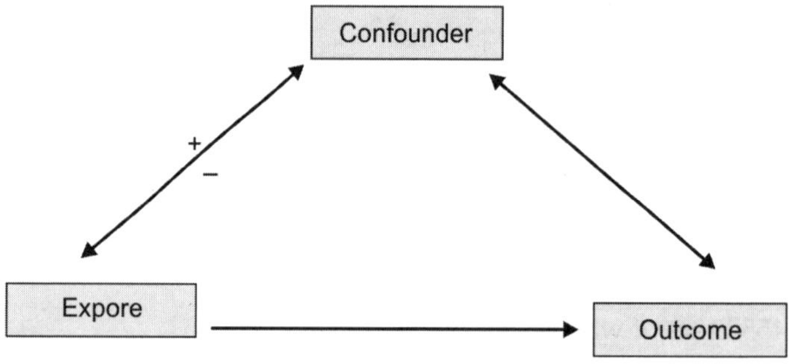

Confounder

Confounder is a factor independently related to both exposure and outcome but unequally distributed among individuals.

Rate

Time specified
Multiplier
Numerator/Denominator
Actual cases/potential cases

Ratio

Between two random variables

Proportion

Numerator is a part of denominator

Before test

$$\text{Senstivity (SN)} = \frac{a}{a+c} \times 100 \text{ (or) } \frac{TP^{\text{(Always truth on top)}}}{TP + FN}$$

$$\text{Specificity (SP)} = \frac{d}{b+d} \times 100 \text{ (or) } \frac{TN}{TN + FP}$$

After test

$$\text{Positive Predictive Value (PPV)} = \frac{a}{a+b} \times 100 \text{ (or) } \frac{TP}{TP + FP} \text{ (all positive)}$$

$$\text{Negative Predictive Value (NPV)} = \frac{d}{c+d} \times 100 \text{ (or) } \frac{FN}{FN + TN} \text{ (all negative)}$$

$1 - \alpha$ = Specificity

$1 - \beta$ = Power of the test = sensitivity

PPV = Diagnostic power of the test

<u>LR</u> (No change with prevalence)

$$\text{Likelihood ratio of Positive test} = \frac{SN}{1\text{–}SP}$$

$$\text{Likelhood ratio of Negative test} = \frac{1\text{–}SN}{SP}$$

Post-test probability = Pretest probability × LR

$$PPV = \frac{P \times SN}{P \times SN + (1 - P)(1 - SP)}$$

$$NPV = \frac{1 - P \times SP}{(1 - P) \times SP + P(1 - SN)}$$

Degree of freedom = (Row – 1) × (Column – 1)

False Positive rate = 1 – specificity (α)

False Negative rate = 1 sensitivity (β)

$$\text{False discovery rate} = \frac{FP}{FP + TP}$$

$$\text{False omission rate} = \frac{FN}{FN + TW}$$

$$\text{Accuracy} = \frac{TP + TN}{TP + TN + FP + FN}$$

$$Z = \frac{x - \bar{x}}{\sigma}$$

σ – Standard deviation

μ – Mean

η – No. of entries

$$\text{Standard Deviation SD} = \sqrt{\frac{\Sigma(x - \bar{x})^2}{n}} = \sqrt{\text{Variance}}$$

$$\text{Coefficient of variation} = \frac{\sigma}{\mu} \times 100$$

Std. error of mean = $\frac{\sigma}{\sqrt{n}}$

Precision = $\frac{\sqrt{n}}{\sigma}$

Correlation coefficient = 100 r^2

Confidence Interval/Limit: = $\mu \pm z \times SE$

or

CI α $\frac{1}{\text{sample size}}$ Sample mean ± $\frac{x-\bar{x}}{\sigma} \times \frac{\sigma}{\sqrt{n}}$

α $\frac{1}{\text{Precision}}$

α Variability

α Confidence level

α Margin of error

α Z scope

Narrow CI is good

If confidence interval in relative risk includes 1 - then it is insignificant to reject the hypothesis

SPM Diagram

Stastistics

Normal Distribution

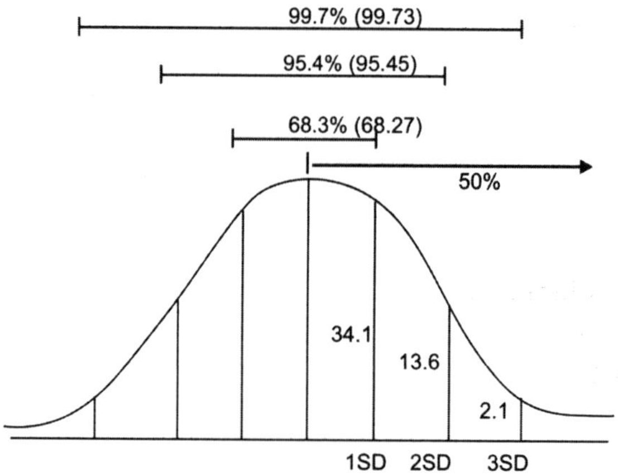

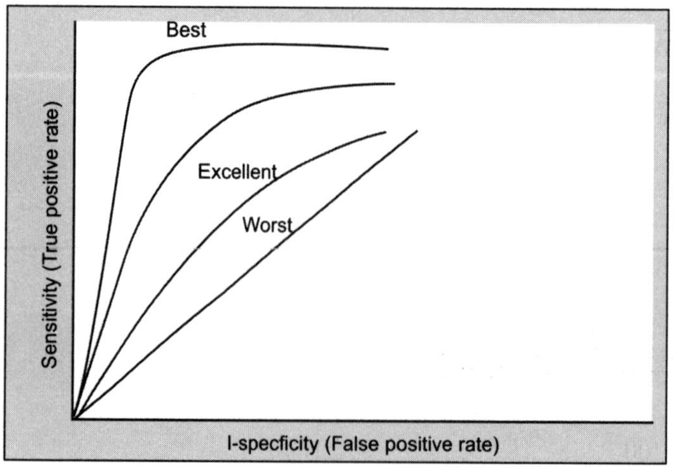

Sample size

Sample size α power of the study

α Std deviation

α loss difference between groups

$$\alpha \frac{1}{\text{P value}} \left(\frac{1}{\alpha}\right)$$

α tailed $\rightarrow$ 2 tailed

$$\frac{\text{Relative risk}}{\text{(for strength of association)}} = \text{RR} = \frac{\text{I (E)}}{\text{I (NE)}}$$

$$\frac{\text{Relative Risk Reduction}}{\text{RRR} = \frac{\text{I (NE)} - \text{I (E)}}{\text{I (NE)}}}$$

Or

$$\frac{\text{ARR}}{\text{I (NE)}}$$

Attributable Risk (For public health)

$$\text{AR} = \frac{\text{I (E)} - \text{I (NE)}}{\text{I (E)}} \times 100$$

Attributable Risk Reduction

ARRR = I (NE) – N (E)

Odds ratio [cross product ratio]

In case control studies incidence cannot be measured, so relative risk cannot be calculated instead

$$\text{Odds ratio} = \frac{\text{Odds of exposed}}{\text{Odds of unexposed}} = \frac{a}{\cancel{a} + b} \Big/ \frac{c}{\cancel{c} + d}$$

Considering 'a' and 'c' negligible when compared to b and d respectively

$$\text{OR} = \frac{a}{b} \Big/ \frac{c}{d} = \frac{ad}{bc}$$

Chi square – Cross-sectional studies

RR – Cohort

Odds ratio – Case control

ARR, RRR – RCT

NPV, PPV – Cross-sectional studies

SN, SP – Case control studies

Population Attributable Risk

$$\text{PAR} = \frac{\text{I (population)} - \text{I (NE)}}{\text{IC (population)}}$$

Number Need to Treat

$$\text{NNT} = \frac{1}{\text{ARR}} = \frac{1}{\text{I(NE)} - \text{I(E)}}$$

Rates:

1. Crude mortality rate = $\frac{\text{No. of deaths}}{\text{Population}}$
2. Cause-specific mortality rate = $\frac{\text{No. of deaths from cause}}{\text{Population}}$

3. Case fatality rate = $$\frac{\text{No. of deaths from cause}}{\text{No. of persons with disease/cause}}$$

4. Proportionate Mortality Rate = $$\frac{\text{No. of deaths from cause}}{\text{All deaths}}$$

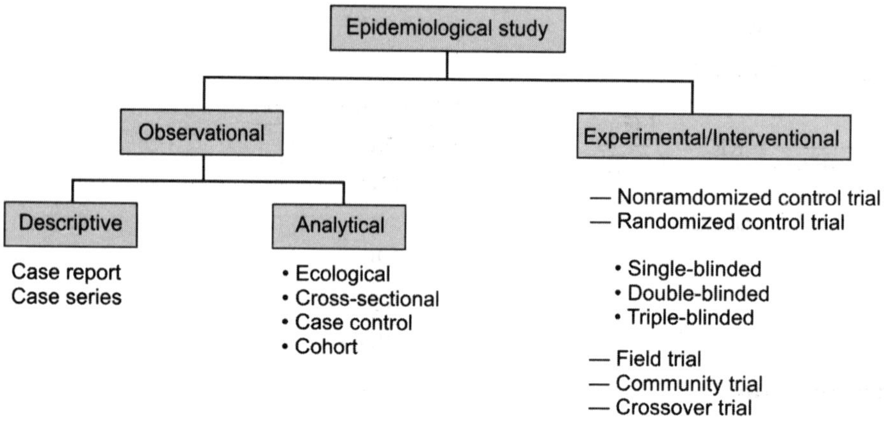